"When someone is brave enough to tell the gritty truth about her tough and twisted journey to self-love and health, you simply have to love her for the forthrightness. But when the writing is this good, and the practical lessons are so transferable, you just count yourself lucky to have discovered her."

—Kathy Freston, *New York Times* bestselling author of *The Lean*

"Jasmin Singer's relentlessly honest memoir is a must-read for anyone who wants to lose that extra 5, 10, 20, or 50 pounds."

—Jane Velez-Mitchell, *New York Times* bestselling author of *iWant*

"[A] moving account of Jasmin's journey to reshaping both body and spirit."

—Neal Barnard, MD, *New York Times* bestselling author of *Power Foods for the Brain*

"A powerful book about a person who comes to self-realization through empathy with others."

—Ingrid Newkirk, president of People for the Ethical Treatment of Animals

"[A] poignant, powerful memoir that is both engaging and enlightening . . . Readers from all walks of life can benefit from reading this book, and will be entertained in the process."

—Melanie Joy, PhD, author of *Why We Love Dogs, Eat Pigs, and Wear Cows: An Introduction to Carnism*

"[Singer's] 'before' and 'after' experiences, told with wisdom and humor, offer a window into the emotional, psychological, social, and commercial factors that complicate our relationship to food and to our bodies." —Joe Cross, filmmaker of *Fat, Sick & Nearly Dead*

"Jasmin Singer is bright and quick and articulate . . . [She] is the real deal. People deserve to read what she has to say."

—Victoria Moran, author of *The Good Karma Diet*

continued . . .

"Gripping, heartfelt, and inspirational."

—Robert Ostfeld, MD, MS, director of the
Cardiac Wellness Program at Montefiore Medical Center

"[A] book that has the power to reach people and to change the world."   —Gene Baur, author of *Living the Farm Sanctuary Life*

"[Singer's] views on food, diet, ethics, and animals will make you think, but more importantly, they will make you act."

—Nathan Runkle, executive director of Mercy for Animals

"[A] tough, poignant, and admirable testimony, one that is bound to inspire a sense of resilience and self-worth among its lucky readers."

—Gena Hamshaw, author of *Choosing Raw*

"An extraordinarily insightful, self-reflective, empathic, and deeply moving memoir . . . This book is as engrossing as it is illuminating."

—Sherry Colb, author of *Mind If I Order the Cheeseburger?*

"[A] coming-of-age story for anyone who has ever questioned both whether they belong and whether they really want to . . . [A] writer you will want to keep your eye on."

—Charles Siebert, author of *The Wauchula Woods Accord*

"Singer tells a deeply personal story with an honesty that is courageous and eloquent, all the while sparkling with humor and intelligence. This is a lovely, memorable, and inspiring book."

—Robin Lamont, author of *The Chain*

"An unflinchingly honest and quirky coming-of-age tale . . . Alternately painful and thrillingly joyous, as Jasmin tells her truth with clarity and grace and biting humor, and a fierce feminist thread running through it all."

—Beth Greenfield, author of *Ten Minutes from Home*

always
too
much
and
never
enough

———

JASMIN SINGER

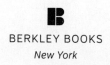

BERKLEY BOOKS

New York

BERKLEY

An imprint of Penguin Random House LLC
375 Hudson Street, New York, New York 10014

Library of Congress Cataloging-in-Publication Data

Names: Singer, Jasmin.
Title: Always too much and never enough : a memoir / Jasmin Singer.
Description: New York : Berkley Books, [2016]
Identifiers: LCCN 2015031565 | ISBN 9780425279571 (paperback)
Subjects: LCSH: Singer, Jasmin—Health. | Overweight persons—Biography. |
Weight loss. | BISAC: BIOGRAPHY & AUTOBIOGRAPHY / Personal Memoirs. |
BIOGRAPHY & AUTOBIOGRAPHY / Women. | COOKING / Vegetarian & Vegan.
Classification: LCC RC628 .S56 2016 | DDC 616.3/980092—dc23 LC record available at
https://lccn.loc.gov/2015031565

PUBLISHING HISTORY
Berkley trade paperback edition / February 2016

PRINTED IN THE UNITED STATES OF AMERICA

10 9 8 7 6 5 4 3 2 1

Cover design by Danielle Abbiate.
Interior text design by Kelly Lipovich.
Interior photo: *JasminAfter* © by Jessica Mahady.

Penguin is committed to publishing works of quality and integrity.
In that spirit, we are proud to offer this book to our readers;
however, the story, the experiences, and the words
are the author's alone.

Penguin
Random
House

Some names and identifying details have been changed to protect the privacy of the famished, the foolish, the bullies, and the bullied.

CONTENTS

CONTENTS

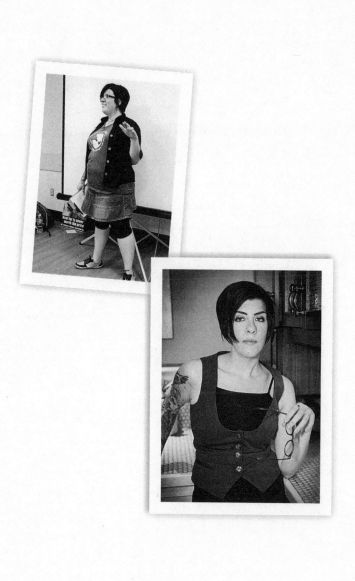

I

what i lost

ONE

---

let's do this

That bathroom stall was ridiculously small. I wriggled my way around, trying to wedge both me and my stupid, gigantic purse into the cramped rectangle. I shimmied, did a tiny pirouette, and finally edged my pants down. It was like *Swan Lake* in there, and all so that I could successfully maneuver my 221-pound, five-foot-four self into proper peeing position.

"This is like a goddamn gestation crate," I said to no one in particular, finally finding a suitable stance, but only after banging my funny bone on the sanitary napkin disposal.

A few minutes later, as small beads of sweat collected on my forehead, I washed my hands, thinking, "Why is soap in public bathrooms always hot pink?"

I was winded. I decided to take a moment to catch my breath. My dining mates could wait. They were probably in a tabbouleh daze by now anyway, busy working their way through the fava bean appetizer.

Oh, how I loved the food in San Francisco! Even in comparison to my own gritty city, New York—which was just bursting with flavors and cuisines vibrant and diverse enough to keep any foodie busy (including a vegan one, like me)—there was something about this town that made me hungry to try everything. On that night, my partner, Mariann, and I had met up with a couple of friends who knew the ins and outs of the restaurant scene in the City by the Bay. They'd chosen a slightly gaudy, but nonetheless mouthwatering, Mediterranean restaurant in the Tenderloin district—ironic, because we were there for its scrumptious vegan menu. The only tenderloins in our lives were made out of wheat gluten.

Just before I excused myself to go to the bathroom, my friends John and Cassie had been telling Mariann and me (but mainly me) about a new documentary, *Fat, Sick & Nearly Dead*, set to be released the following spring. John and Cassie worked in magazine publishing and had been given an advance press copy.

They told us that the film was about a man who juice fasted for sixty days in an effort to get his health back. As he flooded his body with fruits and vegetables, he lost a tremendous amount of weight, got off all his medications, and cured a debilitating autoimmune disease that had plagued him for years. "You really should borrow it, Jasmin," John told me, a bit too adamantly for my taste. "Seriously, you've got to see it."

I fake smiled. "You know what?" I announced. "Nature calls . . ."

The truth is, when John—a naturally excited guy—shared his enthusiasm with me, I took it personally. Was his exuberance a way of calling me fat? Was he comparing me to the man in the film? When I was a kid, I had been accused of making everything about me, and perhaps there was legitimacy in that still. But this hit pretty close to home.

There I was, hiding away in the maroon and turquoise bathroom instead of sitting beside my girlfriend enjoying the company of my good buddies and eating incredible food. I suddenly felt a twinge in my right shoulder. "Dang purse," I mumbled, shaking off the pain. What the hell was I carrying with me, anyway? I opened it up and instantly spotted the culprit: my new shoes.

And by new, I mean old. I had picked up those adorable green and white hemp sneakers at my favorite thrift store in the Mission District earlier that day. I'd forgotten putting them in my bag. Satisfied that I wasn't suddenly suffering from brittle bones, I fished out a lip gloss.

And then, unthinkingly—before having the foresight to prepare myself—I foolishly looked at myself in the mirror.

It's amazing, really, how easy it is to master the art of looking in the mirror without actually looking at yourself—in a way that doesn't make you want to step in front of a bus, that is. I knew all the tricks: how to hang mirrors a few inches too high so my view of myself was always from the way-more-flattering angle above; how to suck in my cheeks just a little bit to give myself fake cheekbones, widening my eyes at the same time to add to the effect; and, finally, how to look at only one part of my body at a time— my eyes if I was putting on shadow, the crown of my head if I was brushing my hair.

Even a simple act like walking down the street with a friend was like a real-life video game. The challenge? To keep the conversation going while avoiding, at all costs, catching a glimpse of my reflection in a window—an image that echoed the truth in ways I was not prepared to handle. And so, rather than take the chance of spotting my silhouette, I would maintain unrelenting eye contact with my hapless companion, who was no doubt wondering why I seemed to be trying to peer into his or her soul. Anything to avert my eyes from the truth, to remain in the dark.

It had been a good number of years, in fact, since I had looked at myself, head-on, in full, with no preparation—with no absurd rationalization of what I was about to see, of *who* I was about to see.

Except, this time, I acted too quickly and, as I stared at myself in the bathroom mirror, I accidentally saw it all: my three chins, my blazer that didn't close, and my Humpty Dumpty figure. Just like that, there I was, without my mirror-face on to protect me.

I was alone in the bathroom, with only myself and my cracked veneer, and yet I was self-conscious, somehow feeling as if I were being watched. My stomach ached, and not because of the numerous triangles of perfectly browned pita bread I'd just eaten. I needed an escape, fast. Just as it started to dawn on me that the intensity I was feeling was my own DIY wall of denial beginning to crumble, I randomly spotted a plastic earring on the floor that someone must have dropped. That one-earringed person was clearly my angel, because in that moment, that plastic earring saved my life—or at least my evening—giving me the distraction I needed to pull myself together.

"Stop feeling sorry for yourself," I quietly commanded. Self-pity was simply not an option. Wallowing should be reserved for people who were truly without. I had no right to be upset just because I was *fat*.

"Focus on what you've got right," I whispered. Like my thick-framed blue and white glasses, which I had bought at Fabulous Fanny's in the East Village, or the two dozen glittery barrettes that decorated my spiky black and pink hair. I had "a look"—that was what people had told me my whole life—and as my weight stepped up, so did my many ornaments. I had always assumed that my eyeliner diverted attention from my bulbous belly and that my nose hoop distracted from my self-consciousness.

And yet, in spite of the temporary respite provided by the lost earring and my standard pep talk, all my warts were still right there, smack in front of me, staring back. At that moment, a familiar, happy thought occurred to me: I was fairly certain that the overwhelming sense of despair that was always lying dormant in me, and that was starting to bubble up right at that instant in the ostentatious bathroom in the Tenderloin, would be effectively cured by spinach pie.

So I put on lip gloss without watching and headed back to my booth, where the all-knowing Mariann shot me the "is everything okay?" look, and I smiled another fake smile—all the while knowing she wouldn't buy the bullshit and we'd have to hash it out later. She was, after all, one of the realest parts of my life—the part that grounded me when the whole world seemed out of control.

"There was a wait," I lied, a little too exuberantly.

And then—Jesus Christ!—it was as though my dining mates had paused the clock and stared into space while I was in the bathroom, counting the seconds until I returned to the booth just to pick up the conversation exactly where we had left off. My abrupt exit had been dramatic only *to me*. Next time I'd have to try harder.

"So, as I was saying," John said as he wiped a dollop of hummus from the right corner of his lip. "You've gotta see this movie, Jazz."

Cassie agreed. "You've gotta. It's a game changer."

A game changer.

When I stepped onstage for the first time in first grade and realized that I could be anyone in the world up there, and maybe I'd be accepted, because I was good at it, and I could be *someone else* while I was center stage—that was a game changer. When I slept with a woman for the first time, at nineteen, that had been a game changer (especially for my then boyfriend). When I learned, at twenty-four, that the food industry was lying to me, and I went vegan—a decision that shaped me, gave me the kind of fulfillment that many people my age only dreamed of having, and added deep and profound purpose to my life—a game changer indeed. When, at twenty-seven, I met Mariann, and together we decided to try to change the world—*game changer.*

I knew a thing or two about changing the game.

I held my breath, wanting so badly to talk about anything besides a man who was fat and sick and nearly dead. A man to whom my friends were obviously comparing me.

Sometimes change comes merely as a result of hearing something at exactly the right moment. Sometimes, like a pair of perfect hemp sneakers at a secondhand store, you have no idea what's about to enter your life.

Given the conversation about the documentary that my friends insisted I "really had to see," it seemed a remarkable coincidence that I had just read an article about juice fasting and, much to my surprise, had found myself intrigued.

The waiter placed my dish in front of me. "The spinach pie, miss."

My belief that spinach pie would distract me from the thoughts that kept bubbling up proved wrong. In spite of the deliciousness that sat right there in front of me, I could no longer refuse to notice the lingering back and shoulder pain that I felt every morning, the rashes I got on my thighs from flesh rubbing against flesh, the deeply buried sadness and anger that hid behind my days. There were only so many glittery barrettes.

My shoulder twinged again—I was used to being achy. Even though I was only thirty, it was difficult for me to go up a flight of stairs without stopping halfway to rest. Sometimes I stopped in the middle, pretending I needed to adjust the cuff of my jeans, or check a pretend text, just to buy some time before finishing the exhausting trek. Why did I feel like shit all the time? I was young, vegan, and even had a master's in health and healing. And yet, I was digging myself an early grave. It was embarrassing.

Even though I rationalized my weight by saying that my life of abundance—decadent food on a consistent basis, several soy lattes a day, wine each night—was a way to repay myself for the hard work I did, the truth was that I knew I was hurting myself. The even deeper truth was that I was *addicted*, and rationalization is the oldest tool of the addict. Even when the results from my physical came in and I was told, point-blank, that my weight and cholesterol were issues that I needed to pay attention to, I *still* rationalized. They weren't big concerns *yet*, I said, and I'd deal with them if and when they became issues.

As I stared down at my spinach pie, I couldn't help but wonder when exactly that moment would come and I would begin to take responsibility for my health.

Cassie, true to form, was now animatedly discussing the newest cashew cheese to hit the market. It's difficult to find more passionate foodies than a group of vegans. My dining mates and I had seen the dark, early days of bad vegan cheese, so we felt we were allowed a little over-the-top excitement on the matter.

I interrupted. "Hey, you guys?" I said, suddenly self-conscious, yet trying—as always—to seem unflappable. "I think I'll borrow that movie you mentioned, if that's cool. The one about being fat and sick?"

"Yeah, sure!" John beamed. "Pick it up from my office tomorrow."

After I picked up the movie and went back to my hotel room and watched it—immediately, on my laptop, with Mariann beside me—everything came to a head. All of it—the lies, the sadness, the rationalization, the heavy heart, the sometimes misdirected anger at the world and at myself—it all culminated in one surprisingly simple, subtle shrug.

"Let's do this," I said.

In retrospect, I am not sure precisely what I meant by "let's do this." It seems to me I was trying to say, "Let's do a juice fast. Let's lose weight. Let's get healthy."

But by "doing this," I wound up committing to a whole lot more than I'd be able to grasp for years to come, and in some ways am still trying to grasp, and maybe always will be. It took losing nearly one hundred pounds for me to start to understand what I was, in fact, "doing." And perhaps more importantly, what the world was doing to me.

The world was, I would later find out, interested in my size to a much greater degree than had ever occurred to me. Because it was only when I lost the weight and my body suddenly seemed to suit the narrow definition of "acceptable"—*slim, svelte, slight*—that I started to experience what it felt like to be propelled upward by the same society that had previously seemed to prefer that I just disappear.

Prior to that proclamation, "Let's do this," I would have told you that I already had a meaningful understanding of the food I ate and the way it affected me and the way it affected the world. I would have theorized that the reason I had always felt as if I was going up the down staircase was because I was offbeat, or because I was an individual thinker, not because I was fat and therefore deemed unworthy by society; not because I was a food addict who was battling shame issues as steadily as I was battling bullies. I ate and lived in a way that was in harmony with my worldview, and I loved that. That had been good enough for me, until suddenly it wasn't. And when it wasn't anymore, that was when something permanently shifted. That was when it became abundantly clear to me that simply eating in a way that avoided hurting others was never going to be enough if my eating habits were still hurting me.

So when I started shedding the weight and reclaiming my health, it was quite a shock to learn that, in order to truly live genuinely, I had to confront how I had been betrayed by a food industry that relied on my willful ignorance and by a society that relied on my undiscerning willingness to buy into its arbitrary notions of self-worth and beauty.

I see now that it was that dinner with my friends that was the turning point. It was the warm decadence and safe reassurance of the spinach pie—that suddenly didn't seem so safe. It was John's persistent vehemence that I just had to watch that documentary. It was Mariann gently squeezing my knee under the table, reminding me that I wasn't alone, that she was beside me. That this was real. That I was real.

It was standing in a bathroom stall, unable to turn around because the walls were closing in on me. It was accidentally

TWO

—

a private affair

Long before I digested just how deeply food had betrayed me (and, chances are, betrayed you), I considered it a friend. And not just a friend—but a soul companion, a trusted confidant. It wooed me, then saved me. (Or so I told myself.)

But then food ruined me. I began to obsessively lust after it, following it, against my better judgment, into dark alleyways and seedy corners. It was the stuff horror movies were made of: the unsuspecting, hungry dame (me) and the ill-intentioned, charming villain (my lunch).

Food was my guru, my lover, my sage. It seduced and defined me. And, ultimately, it deceived me.

There was a time, however, when it simply fed me.

I was completely ordinary, for the first and final time, when I was a little tiny kid living in the circle-shaped condo development known as Pumptown Corners, nestled in a small Anytown, U.S.A., called Edison, New Jersey. What I wore, who I loved, and what I ate were about as normal as blueberry pie.

Every activity in which I partook, every hobby I embraced, every passion I fostered, and every Slurpee I slurped was exactly what you'd imagine a middle-class suburban girl in the 1980s would spend her time obsessing about. On the weekends, I would wake up to the sweet smell of not-so-homemade Bisquick pancakes—my favorite—with margarine and without the gooey syrup I couldn't stand. I'd carefully cut my two perfectly circular and lightly browned pancakes into small, soft triangles, and, as I dangled my bare feet beneath me and hummed the theme to *General Hospital*, I'd take a few satisfying bites, then quickly throw on my tutu just in time to rush to the ballet class I took at the nearby university. My mother, a stunningly beautiful, svelte artist with a fervent love of fashion and a talent for preparing prepackaged food that had me thinking she was the next Chef Boyardee, would drop me off for my little kid lessons in how to plié.

My brother, Jeremy—four years my senior—was obsessed with the New York Mets (the eighties was a good time for that), and everything in his bedroom was blue and orange. We argued incessantly, eighties-style: I wanted to watch *My Little Pony* and he wanted to watch *Knight Rider.* I wanted to play Candy Land and he wanted to play Connect Four. I wanted elbow macaroni with margarine for dinner and he wanted pastina with cheese. Still, despite our sibling rivalry, Jeremy and I bonded over Twix bars, Nok Hockey, self-recorded radio shows, and watching the brand-new TV station known to the rad kids as MTV. Much of the music played on it was too old for me, but I longed for my brother's maturity and the "big kid" attention it got him, so I sat beside him while he sang all the words to videos like Tom Petty's "Don't Come Around Here No More." I was fascinated by the giant, life-sized Alice in Wonderland cake memorialized in the video and often dreamed of Mom making one for a special occasion. Surely there was a cake mix for that. I wholeheartedly believed in Mom's mixing skills.

The place we hung our Mets hats was forty-five minutes and a whole world away from New York, home to big fat pretzels with thick pebbles of salt just waiting to be licked off; we always picked these up first thing whenever we'd drive in to see a Broadway show, the absolute highlight of my rather idyllic existence.

In Pumptown, my best friend, Tamika, lived only a short bike ride away. When I stayed over at her house, her much older and wiser sister let us stay up to watch *Saturday Night Live*. The humor of it went completely above our heads, but we felt so cool being awake at eleven thirty that it didn't matter. We designated her parents' walk-in closet as our "clubhouse," and we'd hold important meetings that consisted solely of eating entire rows of crunchy Chips Ahoy.

Everything was charmingly normal. I was a freckle-faced brunette with crooked bangs and a side ponytail that sat sloppily atop my head. Punky Brewster was my style icon (admittedly, she might still be . . .) and my self-chosen wardrobe consisted of what were to me thoroughly fashion-forward outfits ranging from a well-worn Strawberry Shortcake dress that Mom scored at a garage sale to bright fluorescent, purposefully paint-splattered T-shirts paired with shiny, hot pink spandex leggings.

Most weekends, Grandma and Grandpa would come over—an event I looked forward to with a monomaniacal intensity that surpassed even my deep fascination with Dr. Brown's celery soda, Grandma's go-to soft drink. I was certain that the highlight of

Grandma and Grandpa's week was seeing me, too, because when they walked in the door (six-pack of celery soda in hand), their eyes lit up, and they were instantly dying to know everything new about our worlds. I felt it was my duty not to leave any detail unreported, so I would sit on Grandpa's lap or cuddle in Grandma's warm, soft arms, and update them on what had happened that week on *Family Ties*, or the latest knock-knock joke I had learned from my ever-growing collection of joke books. They listened intently, asking the right questions, nodding at the right moments, and laughing with the perfect pitch of enthusiasm.

Grandma and I, in particular, had a deep connection that convinced me that soul mates are not reserved solely for romance. My very first memory is with Grandma—just sitting with her on a sunny day, on the back porch—and the overarching theme of that memory, and of all my memories with her, is that of safety. Her warm arms were safe. Her pastel house was safe. Talking to her was safe, free of judgment and mental clutter. Her love was dependable. It remained that way until the very end, and somehow—even though she died when I was thirty-four, leaving a gaping hole in my heart and my life—her love still gives me a sense of sanctuary. I clung to that as a child, when the whole world felt broken and upside down, and I still cling to it.

Grandpa, always the jolly, soft-spoken do-gooder, briefly had a volunteer job taking low-income people who didn't drive to their jobs, and so he had access to this enormous van—the perfect vehicle to take my entire family out for ice cream sundaes in style. I'd get chocolate everything—chocolate ice cream, chocolate sprinkles, chocolate syrup—always in a cup, never a messy, breakable, undependable cone. I'd savor tiny bites and imagine that this was probably how Duran Duran felt all the time as I gazed out the window at my impressive wheels—and then I'd glance at my vanilla-mouthed grandpa, the chauffeur, who knew exactly how to make a four-year-old feel like the most special girl in the world.

My mother and father had gotten divorced, after being married for seven grueling years, when I was a year old and Jeremy was five. Their divorce was ugly and complicated, and now, thirty-five years later, it still is. My father was a charismatic and emotional man—a talented musician who insisted on being the center of attention whether he was at a small family get-together or a large-scale party. With him, everything was black or white, one extreme or the other, including people's opinions of him.

Though my parents' divorce was hostile, and tension from it ran like a low-lying electrical current throughout my childhood, even as a kid I knew that I was somehow lucky not to remember what it was like when they were a couple, as my brother did. We were often thrust into the middle of ongoing battles that my parents should have worked out in private, but the stories that circulated in my family about their screaming fights were haunting. I am sure that my brother's firsthand recollections of them, as a young child, were scarring, and quite possibly the reason why he went through school with frequent suspensions and detentions. He was always getting into trouble.

I, on the other hand, at least in those early, idyllic years, was a well-behaved, easygoing child. After the divorce, we lived with Grandma and Grandpa for a while until my mother met Brock, my first stepfather. Brock represented everything that Dad did not:

patience, even-temperedness, and gentleness. Brock—a divorced man himself, with a daughter just older than Jeremy—was an English professor, banjo player, and train trivia expert. Mom and Brock had only been dating briefly when they decided to get married—an impulsive decision Mom probably made in hopes that Brock would provide the emotional stability that my father didn't, and that my and Jeremy's childhood frequently lacked.

That is when we moved to Pumptown—my flailing mother in search of consistency, my Mets-obsessed brother in search of home base, and me innocently in search of red Skittles. For a very brief time, we all found what we needed. Pumptown was normal; our life was easy. Mom promptly commemorated our new beginning by painting an enormous wall that ran beside our split-level stairs with a colorful and bold sunrise.

Brock was a caring and fun-loving stepfather. My early childhood memories of him are all tender and sweet. He and Mom had a nightly ritual of interlocking their hands, chairlike, and carrying me to my room, where they'd swing me onto my bed as I giggled uncontrollably and begged them to do it again. In Pumptown, my ballet lessons kept me busy, my Bisquick kept me fed, and my family kept me happy.

Sadly for me, their marriage, lackluster and passionless, lasted less than two years. From my point of view, their marriage couldn't have been better: Brock made an excellent stepfather. I was comfortable around him and often found solace simply sharing space in the room with him while we each busied ourselves with our own activities. He would sit cross-legged on the armchair and read the paper and I would sprawl nearby on the floor and play with my My Little Pony collection, my Legos, or my M&M's. It was a six-year-old's dream.

We were both at the kitchen table—me propped up a little by the phone book booster seat and Brock beside me—when I taught myself how to multiply by strategically placing my M&M's in rows. "Brock, is three times three nine?" I asked, wide-eyed, as I stared at my multicolored chocolate-shelled masterpiece. Brock was wildly impressed by my findings, and his exuberant validation resulted in an ear-to-ear smile that I could not shake for days. (I always knew that M&M's were magical.)

When Mom and Brock decided to call it a day, Mom couldn't stomach the task of breaking my heart, and so it was Brock who was saddled with the thankless job of telling me that their marriage had fallen apart. He sat me down on the big brown corduroy armchair in their bedroom—a resilient chair that later followed me to each of my many Manhattan apartments throughout my twenties.

He knelt down and I could see the big hairless circle on top of his head. "Your mom and I are splitting up, Jazz," he whisper-said, and I remember feeling like I was kicked in the stomach, then promptly reminding myself that *breaking up is just what adults do.* I didn't protest; I simply hung my head in defeat and stared down at my lap, bit my lower lip, clutched at the material of my Strawberry Shortcake dress, and let sadness and confusion dull my fluorescence. Turned out that corduroy chair was more resilient than I was.

Just like that, Brock was gone, and Mom was single again. Pumptown Corners lost some of its sparkle, and a new emptiness seeped its way into my days.

Still, despite the rockiness of her relationships with men, my mother's love for Jeremy and me was consistent and all encompassing. Though it was my grandmother who provided me with steadiness, taught me about unconditional adoration in the very special way that only grandmas can perfect, and allowed me to eat all the chocolate-covered jelly rings I could manage, Mom was a solid force. She did not always have it easy—and yet she constantly put us ahead of everything else. Perhaps she did so to a flawed degree, but she was wild about us and always made sure to provide us with support and compassion.

When she was newly divorced from Brock, Mom took Jeremy and me on vacation. In my memory, we were living it up in the lap of luxury—playing board games, going hiking, eating American cheese sandwiches on soft bread, acting out funny characters that Mom constantly created in order to keep us entertained. I was an adult before I found out Mom's version of that trip: that the only thing she could afford was to take us to stay at a rustic cabin at a Boy Scout camp, off-season, and the whole place was filthy, bug infested, and nonfunctional. She later told me about how she carried me on her back up the barn ladder that led to the sleeping area, then draped clean blankets all over the muddy, splintery floor. I didn't remember any of that—I only remembered being absolutely ecstatic about having my mom and brother all to myself, in this mystical place that was apparently falling to pieces around me without me noticing.

Perhaps there's validity to my memory of this trip being better than it actually was—I had my family to myself, which was all that mattered to me at the time—while my struggling mother remembers it as much worse. Someplace in the middle of those two memories is the truth, suspended somewhere in the mid-1980s like Punky Brewster's messy pigtails, never to be untangled.

When we returned from our luxury vacation, I felt the absence of Brock, and of life-as-I-knew-it. In school, I longed for my moody second-grade teacher, Mrs. Poppet, to take notice and ask me what was wrong. I certainly wouldn't have known how to answer, but I craved the question. Moodiness aside, she was, after all, a mother herself, so didn't that make her a parental figure by default? I wanted an adult, maternal or not, to simply acknowledge my reality, that things had shifted for me in a big way.

One day, I convinced myself that if I scribbled nonsensically on my assignment, Mrs. Poppet would remove her permanent frown long enough to become concerned with my uncharacteristic gibberish, and she'd gently pull me over to the side to say, "Honey, is everything okay?"

Of course, that was not at all what happened. Instead, I got reprimanded for not following the rules and for "ruining a perfectly nice ditto." I was given a second chance at the assignment. Sure that if I scribbled on it yet again Mrs. Poppet would get the hint, I tried the same trick a second time. This time, she became thoroughly exasperated, and so I was taken out of my class altogether and permanently placed in another one, where a different teacher could be saddled with my rebellious ways. So much for manipulation tactics. I forgot about my sadness and my need for attention when, on the first day in my new class, we made homemade butter and then promptly consumed it on crunchy French bread. It seemed I had struck gold. Two points for manipulation tactics.

I recently recounted this story to my mother, since, even in its retelling now, it seems to be missing a piece. What teacher would simply switch a seven-year-old student to another class for acting out in this relatively benign way? "I remember you switched classes," Mom responded, when I brought it up to her, "but I don't remember anything about scribbling on the report. The class change was, as I recall, due to a personality conflict between you and your teacher."

Which begs the question: Why did anyone, least of all my mother, think it was normal for a teacher to have a "personality conflict" with a second grader? Changing classrooms changed my entire life in drastic ways, and yet the adults just didn't seem to notice that I might be perplexed and even infuriated. So I did what kids everywhere do when their lives turn upside down: I sucked it up and mindlessly swallowed the new normal. With that, and just as mindlessly, I swallowed the bites of bread and butter that my new teacher, Mrs. Jones, foisted upon me with a smile and a wink. That wink seemed to say, "This will make it better." And, like magic, it did.

There were a few other wrinkles that needed smoothing over as well. My mother and father were in a constant court battle for child support (Dad was consistently late with payments, sometimes not paying altogether), and neither of them shielded my brother and me from their explanations of exactly why he or she was right, and why the other was a despicable human being who was unworthy of our devotion. Alternate weekends with my father were tense for me. There was never a comfortable accommodation for us in his house, and my mother and father differed so drastically in terms of parenting techniques that the excessive freedom I was given when I was with him (compared to the limits set by my overprotective mother) was jarring.

During one weekend trip to an amusement park town, Wildwood, my father let me and Jeremy go off by ourselves and told us to meet him back at the hotel later that night. The fact was he was probably going off to get a drink—or, more likely, several. Jeremy, annoyed by his pestering little sister, left me so that he could go ride some big-kid roller coasters. I somehow found my way back to the hotel and to our room, but then stayed up all night literally shaking with fear. I got through the night by closing my eyes tight and imagining my grandmother's arms wrapped around me.

Meanwhile, Mom moved on again. By the time she met Wayne, a quiet and tolerant engineer with a PhD that he never mentioned, who didn't own one pair of jeans (until my mother took him shopping), "divorce" and "remarriage" were becoming two very common words in my vocabulary.

Dad was also busy expanding my ever-growing roster of parents. He had recently gotten remarried to Muriel, a fiery and smart woman who zealously loved cats. Every present she gave me throughout the few years of their marriage was somehow feline themed—books about kittens, cat stuffed animals, sweatshirts with kitty ear patterns. She even baked cat-shaped sugar cookies, which I ate exuberantly. Muriel often told me she thought I was the cat's meow.

I guess I thought that having multiple parents was simply part of growing up, as common as Cabbage Patch dolls (mine was named Casey and had red hair to match Grandma's). The day Jeremy and I waited to meet Wayne, who would become our permanent stepfather, though we didn't know it yet, we busied ourselves playing Nok Hockey in the finished basement at Pumptown Corners. "I'm nervous," I told him. I was seven.

Jeremy sneered. "Why? It's just another one of Mom's dumb boyfriends." He then aggressively scored a goal while I was lost in thought—busy contemplating whether I should change into my Strawberry Shortcake dress, by now slightly too small for me but which I had already worn three times that week anyway. I decided against it, instead stopping our game early in order to grab a fistful of buttered popcorn that Jeremy had just microwaved—the perfect salty distraction.

A half hour and second bag of microwaved popcorn later, a tall, handsome-in-a-nerdy-way man, with a beard and mustache that hid his mouth almost completely, descended the basement stairs—and immediately demonstrated his good sense by presenting me with a ceramic clown doll, which to this day sits on my windowsill.

It was decided soon after that Mom and Wayne would get married and we would leave Pumptown Corners for yet another fresh start. I took one last look at my bedroom with the rainbow decal plastered onto the pink wall, and I cried inconsolably. Tears streaming, I rode my bike to Tamika's house for the final time and told her I'd see her around. We ate cookies in silence and sadness. It was our Last Supper. We decided to memorialize the moment by giving ourselves tiny cuts on our fingers and rubbing the wounds together—"Blood sisters for life," we whispered—and we agreed to continue to stay up late, even by ourselves, and watch *Saturday Night Live*.

I left Tamika's with a stinging cut on my finger and a gnawing sense that the safety of Pumptown would never be replicated anywhere else. When I returned home with a puffy face, I found Mom and Wayne busy rolling white paint all over our beloved sunrise mural that decorated the big wall by the stairs, an image that just a few years prior had been symbolic of our fresh, sunny beginning. I secretly stood at the foot of the stairs and watched as the vibrant orange sun and its bright yellow rays disappeared. The wall was a grayish white now. It didn't belong to us anymore. Pumptown was slipping away, just as Brock had. The sun was gone and, though I didn't know it at the time, the chill I felt should have warned me that for whatever reason, my brief fling with feeling "normal" was over, too. I wouldn't get it back for a long time.

The following week, we moved to Anna Lane, to a yellow house with white shutters, on a freshly paved cul-de-sac, in a different part of Edison, with a different school. On the day we moved in, the four of us sat around a sturdy cardboard box in our new kitchen—we hadn't yet located the table—and brought in an extra-large double cheese pizza. It had been a long day of moving, and we were all hungry. As I sat dangly legged on a flimsy folding chair, surrounded by a new iteration of my family, I rubbed my thumb over the spot on my pointer finger that I had pricked when Tamika and I became blood sisters just the week before. The spot was completely healed, which saddened me.

I could practically taste the absence of Tamika, and of the rest of my life that I had known so well. Suddenly, I became panic-stricken that I wouldn't fit in anymore—a fear that wound up coming true, in spades. The safety of Pumptown was gone, I had officially outgrown my beloved Strawberry Shortcake dress, and even though I wasn't yet eight years old, the newly formed chip on my shoulder made it clear that I was no longer a little kid.

My family all stared at me as I grabbed a third, and then a fourth piece of pizza.

I was, I realized then, absolutely ravenous.

It's amazing how clearly I remember that hot and crunchy pizza from thirty years ago. I see now that food, and the comfort it carried, had been slowly inching its way up in value for me, culminating in that piece of pie—and in the many other bites that began to etch the lines of my days. Food, up until around that point, had simply been what I ate. It did not yet define me. It did not yet provide me with the close companionship that I desperately craved. It did not yet give me the solace I required after a long day of being the new kid at school. It did not yet provide the relief I needed from gradually coming to feel that I was a circular-shaped peg trying to stuff myself into a tiny square hole. It was not yet my constant distraction, my unconditional source of love, my trusted confidant. Up until our move, food was just food.

That all changed—quickly and furiously—when we drove across town and landed on Anna Lane.

New kid. The very words have the ring of childhood misery. Being one, in the middle of the year in third grade, was not the kind of challenge I was ready for. Cliques had already been formed, the totem pole order of the class established. Looking at the situation from an adult sociological point of view, I suppose that having someone jump into a social group made up of children who are just reaching the age where group dynamics matter and bullying seems like a viable strategy is disorienting, not only for the newcomer, but for the other kids, too, who don't quite know how to make sense of this new variable that's suddenly in their way, taking up their space.

I was not the type of kid who could successfully negotiate this new social setting. I had suddenly become painfully shy, a new trait of mine that manifested when we moved. The other kids thought I was "retarded" because my eyes were so heavy lidded and because I didn't say a word, not to anyone—not even a simple "this is so totally rad" on the much-anticipated "J Day," when we were learning how to write *J* in cursive and everybody had to practice by writing *Jasmin*. I was lonesome, and I longed for my old bedroom with the rainbow decal, the condo with the bright mural on the wall. I ached for familiar comfort.

Thankfully, there was one very obvious place I knew of where I could find that. And so it went that, during a time when I was feeling forlorn and disoriented—years before I deemed it my enemy—food became my new best friend.

The friendship had been forged that first day in the new house with the pizza, when I calmed my stomach and mood with the melty cheese, the thick, crunchy crust, and the feeling of security that can only come from fullness to the point of bursting. In one swift meal, full became my new normal, and I sought it with a fierce fervor. Fullness was reliable, I realized then. I could control it, and each time thereafter that my stomach ached from carrying too much food for one little girl's body, a sense of security and accomplishment spread to my limbs and heart, tingling and satisfying, blanketing me with a staggering sense of order.

Changes at school were simultaneous with big shifts at home, and there were bumpy times there as well. My mother decided that since they were getting married, it made sense for me and Jeremy to start to call Wayne "Dad," even though, of course, we already had one of those (even if she preferred to believe otherwise). I can now see that in her own way, her proclamation that Wayne was now "Dad" was emblematic that she, too, was desperately grasping for a sense of normalcy. But for me, that didn't work. I had to live in my world, not hers, and that world already had a "Dad."

For a while I acquiesced—figuring that Mom knew the rules of having a new family better than most, so calling your stepfather "Dad" surely must be an appropriate gesture. But when Jeremy began to protest Wayne's new label, I followed his lead, feeling what had become a very familiar sensation regardless of which of my angry and very vocal parents I happened to be with: that I somehow needed to come to the alternate parent's defense.

"But we already have a dad!" Jeremy yelled—and I echo-shouted, "Yeah! We already have a dad!" with my little arms crossed and my brow furrowed, proving that I meant business. Mom and Wayne just stared back at us blankly, knowing this was a sinking ship with no life preservers for them.

From that day on, we called Wayne "Wayne." The whole episode left me very uneasy, though, and Wayne became the victim of my angst. Such, I suppose, is the lot of stepparents. Projecting all my problems onto Wayne and acting like a spoiled brat probably started when I sensed Jeremy's frustration with him—a frustration that, in hindsight, I can see was almost certainly unfounded. So I, too, took out my angst and anger on Wayne, rather than on my parents or my classmates, and proceeded to spend the next decade doing everything I could to make him feel like scum.

I was the worst possible stepdaughter you could imagine. I would mumble choice insults at him just loudly enough for him to hear and just quietly enough for nobody else to. I would steal money from his drawer to buy Hershey's bars at the drugstore down the street, mimic him behind his back, and—in what I liked to think of as a unique and creative form of acting out—eat dinner with him at the table only if I was surrounded by a fort of cereal boxes, simply so that I could avoid looking at him and watching him eat. When my mother finally put her foot down and told me that I was no longer allowed to shield my spot with the cereal boxes, I covered my left eye, as if my hand were a visor, and stuck my thumb in my ear, because the last thing in the world I wanted was to hear or see

Wayne consume food. That's not to say Wayne was a gross eater; I simply didn't want to share that space with him and resented that I was being forced to. So, unfortunately for Wayne, I became the rudest and brattiest possible dining companion. Wayne sat on my left, so—even though I'm left-handed—I taught myself how to eat with my right. Anything to keep my dinner a private affair.

My anger at Wayne was unwarranted and unfair—he was, after all, an innocuous guy. More than that, he was good to me—always driving me to my playdates, making sure I had what I needed, and even taking the day off work to join Grandma and watch me in the school spelling bee (he even didn't seem to mind that I was the very first one out, adding an extra *l* to *deliver*). Still, looking back, it doesn't even remotely surprise me that I was desperately seeking a scapegoat—and an escape. I didn't know I was being unfair—I only knew how I felt. And it doesn't surprise me that these feelings reached their apex at the dinner table. For me, the act of eating was deeply intimate and personal—something that remained my own even when nothing else seemed to be—and I had no interest in sharing that activity with someone I had decided to hate. Mealtimes became joyless for my whole family, thanks to me—a time to manage my petulance and frustration.

Yet, through all my acting out, and when practically everyone else felt like my enemy, food replaced Tamika as my best friend for life. It was food and me against the rest of the world, and the rest of the world started with my family.

I found solace not only in being a complete bitch to Wayne, but also in something equally bad for my heart: eating cheese. Lots and lots and lots of cheese. We kept a breadbox stashed with

crackers in the hallway between the front door and the kitchen—
the perfect place for me to grab a box of Cheez-Its or saltines
without anyone noticing so I could bring them upstairs to my
pink, troll-infested bedroom and consume the entire box in blissful peace while watching *Growing Pains* or listening to *A Chorus
Line*. If I was really lucky, and my mother was busy placing a
phone order with QVC, as was her daily habit, I could sneak into
the kitchen and quickly snag the Easy Cheese to create the most
delicious, cute little swirl for my perfect cracker square.

As the year went on and I slowly started to recognize that my
family's makeup was indeed atypical—a reality that slapped me
across the face when my father and Muriel split up, and I knew
I'd never get a worthy cat tchotchke again—I took a step back
and tried to honestly assess my family.

I suppose that becoming more objective about your family is
some kind of normal developmental step. But for me at the time,
that assessment simply revealed the obvious fact that I had an
unusual number of parents. Another fact that I had never before
noticed suddenly became crystal clear to me: My mother was
remarkably beautiful. I began to wonder if I would ever forgive
her for it.

I had always suspected that she was elegant. But, after the first
parent-teacher meeting at my new school, when my fourth-grade
teacher mentioned to me how gorgeous my mother was, I realized
that my hunch was correct. She was not only ravishing, she had
a killer figure, too—and as my teacher's frequent comments about
"what an attractive mother I had" proved, she was a real

head-turner. The great lengths she took to get there should have tipped me off.

Mom's morning routine mystified me. I would often sit on the corner of her bed and watch as she delicately applied her makeup—slightly bronzed cheeks with emphasis to the upper cheekbones; forest green eye shadow with tiny little chestnut brown wings penciled on just above her lash line; rosy lips, precisely lined and filled in like the work of a true artist, which Mom was. She would gently lift and tease her short, stylish auburn hair, and I would silently observe—taking in her precise technique, while mindlessly snacking on a sleeve of saltines as I watched the show unfold before my eyes.

I licked the salty top of a crisp cracker as Mom widened her eyes and applied a dark coat of mascara. I delicately nibbled while Mom just as delicately degunked a corner of her eye. My new grown-up teeth chipped away at the rest of the cracker, going clockwise, while Mom strategically dabbed her grown-up perfume on her pulse points. My cracker was gone, as were Mom's skin blotches—magic!

I didn't know whether I should be proud of my gorgeous mother or ashamed that my own looks paled in comparison. And perhaps most confusing to me was how separated Mom seemed to be from her beauty. She was always unhappy with her reflection, always striving for a perfection she couldn't seem to find. This was especially true when it came to her body, even though to look at her, there was no denying that her figure was what the world considered ideal, the perfect shape to display the most form-fitting fashions.

In a fascinating illustration of simple physics, as Mom—or, as

I liked to refer to her, my "TM," for "Thin Mother"—dieted, I ate more. And as Mom criticized her body, her perfect shape, I began to notice my own imperfect one. I didn't yet hold the deep-seated hatred of my body that would manifest in just a few years, but even as a little girl, I started to wonder why hers was hard and mine soft, her stomach flat and mine lumpy. I didn't understand why she was seemingly satisfied eating a tiny, cardboard-encased diet TV dinner, while my robust blackened cheeseburger with steak fries, and canned peas with margarine (to get my veggies in), was never nearly enough. Add to that my inability to share a normal meal with Wayne, and, in retrospect, I can see the emergence of my convoluted relationship with food and my body. Eating became a private affair for me, as often as I could manage.

That was about the time that I began eating my bagged lunches in the privacy of a bathroom stall at school.

My TM always packed me little notes telling me she loved me and encouraging me to do well that day. And so my reassuring notes and I sat on the toilet lid while I ate our sandwich, which was generally filled with bologna as well as my beloved cheese. Many years later I learned that bologna is a product that the USDA insists must be "comminuted," or reduced to minute particles, so that you can't recognize the flecks of lard in it. You might as well call it "lard paste" and save the term "baloney" for the marketing that convinced my mom that this so-called food would give kids a healthy, compact meal when in fact it probably would have been nutritionally preferable to eat actual paste. But at the time, it was welcome company, comminuted or not.

As I became less the new kid and more just the different one, and my classmates reacted to my presence with a mix of acceptance (not to be confused with approval) and perplexity, I slowly left my shyness behind. By fourth grade, I spoke up when I had things to say. When a newer, younger girl was being teased on the playground, I screamed at the perpetrators and defiantly hung out with the new kid. She appreciated my effort to stand up for her, but soon enough realized that I was a pariah—not the girl you wanted to form your social circle around.

Once uncool, always uncool, and it seemed my reputation preceded me. I was already considered unworthy and unattractive. Damned was the dodgeball team that got me on it—I was their wart, and the other team brought attention to that fact whenever possible.

Food was my salvation and my companion. It was the piece of me that came along when I left Pumptown Corners for Anna Lane. It was an intimate extension of my thoughts, my moods, even my body—Smarties were commonly stuffed into the pockets of my bright orange Windbreaker, Twinkies in the small pocket of my backpack, Twizzlers slipped up my sleeves. Food was safely situated in the cabinets of my father's house when I would sneak into the kitchen late at night. It was scrupulously stocked in the breadbox of my house on Anna Lane, where I could easily and quietly take my share, or more than my share. Food knew me, and knew it had a hold on me.

And in spite of everything else that I was unsure of—my burgeoning body, my unfamiliar family, my unseemly father, my damaged reputation—I knew food.

Oh, how preciously and precisely *I knew food.*

THREE

---

there are no small parts,
only fat actors

I was seriously going to pee in my pants. *Why did I have that extra Coke at lunch?* Something had to be done, or my classmates would have an actual reason to make fun of me. I hesitantly raised my hand, asked to please be excused, then braced myself for the worst eight seconds of my day—the exact amount of time it took for me to walk from my desk to the classroom door.

I stood up, and the first of what would coincidentally be eight insults (one for each second it took me to get to the front) was hurled.

By Margaret. I should have known. Margaret was your classic definition of beautiful—a fact not lost on her, or on any other of my fifteen-year-old classmates. That day, it was she who started the coughing fit—a ritual my classmates reserved just for me—complete with a crescendo of fake throat-clearings that hid inside of them words and phrases like "Fatso," "Fatty," and "Fuck you." Lizzie, Melinda, and Stacey quickly joined in, poorly disguising their insults (cough, cough, *whale* . . . cough, cough, *pig*). Everyone seemed to be in on it—except the teacher, that is, who ignored their taunting, which was easier for him than dealing with it. He kept his head down and his mouth shut as he reviewed the imminent homework assignment—and as I began my walk of shame to the front of the room to grab the bathroom key.

I pretended not to hear them. That was what I was supposed to do. I was still a good kid then, still played by the rules. The rules also said, in bold print, "Don't cry in front of them," and so I didn't.

But inside I screamed. Inside, I took my oversized, underread history textbook and I smacked it clear across Margaret's pretty, petite face.

I reached the front of the room, knowing that this was the moment I was the most exposed. My hair was in two French braids, and my long hippie skirt collected debris at the bottom. "Nice outfit," remarked Sandra—her comment, though clearly sarcastic, was offered in a manner covert enough that it almost vaguely resembled kindness. I looked in her direction, caught a glimpse of her overeager pretend smile. And I thanked her.

By this point, my classmates had long before decided where I stood in the hierarchal order of desirability—namely, the bottom. My freckles had long diminished and my waistline expanded. My crooked bangs grew out and my outcast status settled in. Like other teenagers, I adored getting new outfits, and yet shopping had become a frustrating and disheartening activity. At size fourteen, standing at five foot two, for me the Juniors section was simply not an option.

Even though that was over twenty years ago, frustratingly, this kind of sizeism continues—alienating heftier girls (and women) by delegating them to the tent section of the department store, where the only "cute" things in their size are often the necklaces and espadrilles. At fifteen—and for a lot of my life—I didn't even have the option of shopping in plus-size stores (and the clothes in the Misses department were more suited for the older ladies Grandma hung out with than for a teen like me). Like so many other girls and women, I was in the dreaded purgatory of an "in-between" size: too voluminous for Juniors, too small for Plus.

Not that my TM would have allowed me to set foot into the Plus department anyway.

We were at Menlo Park Mall when I tried. Though Mom's department of choice for herself was, indeed, Juniors, she understood that my bulbous belly and watermelon-sized breasts were not going to fit into a trendy and figure-hugging slip dress anytime soon. Our shopping expeditions always started in Juniors anyway, which was due more to my own insistence than hers. Though I understood, on some level, that I was much larger than my waif-like, still-gangly peers, I still held out hope that my fatness was my mirror's doing and did not reflect reality.

So Mom and I would venture to the Juniors section of Macy's, where she would inevitably find an adorable, stylish, and arguably too-young-for-her skirt or sweater. I'd pout behind her on line at the checkout, popping bubble gum, staring at the square pattern on the floor, and hiding the sadness on my face with my very long black hair and feigned blasé attitude.

It was one particularly rainy day—I remember that because my raincoat refused to button in the front—when, after Mom's Juniors expedition during a trip to the mall, I noticed a glimmer of hope in the window of Lane Bryant. Lane Bryant was the all-plus-size, all-the-time haven for the humongous among us—a store I had never even noticed before, except for the fact that I regularly passed it on the way to Cinnabon.

For some reason, on this rainy day when my sweatshirt was soaked down the middle, it held my gaze, slowing my pace and quickening my heartbeat. Mom, holding her crisp brown Macy's bag, stopped walking a few steps in front of me when she realized I was distracted by something.

I stared into the store window. The first thing I noticed was that Lane Bryant featured thicker mannequins than its neighbor, the Gap. The second thing I noticed was that those mannequins were wearing slip dresses and short denim vests—exactly the wardrobe popular at my high school, and at virtually every other high school in the United States in 1994.

I looked around to make sure that nobody from my school was nearby. I didn't want to be seen, maybe not even by myself. When the coast was clear, I gathered up my resolve and quickly asked the question that was burning on my tongue. "Mom, can I go in here?"

My TM looked up and saw the store I was referring to—Lane Bryant. A store for fat people, not for your teenage daughter. (Well, not for *her* teenage daughter.) She tried to speak, then choked a little on her saliva—elongating the moment even more. Finally, when she could speak, she said, "Jazz, you're not going to find anything there." Her gaze was still fixed on the store sign—she was clearly a little horrified.

I looked back at the mannequins. I imagined myself wearing those clothes, and again, I felt like maybe I should at least try. They were so much more in style than my hippie skirts and big sweat-shirts. But Mom's reaction hit me in the gut, because even though all she said was that those clothes wouldn't work for me, she couldn't disguise the curtness and the lack of enthusiasm in her tone.

Perhaps she meant for me to hear it. I'm sure that my chubbiness was terrifying to her. She didn't know where to put it, how to rationalize it, or how to fix it. She had been trying time and time again to get me to shed pounds—often bringing me with her to her Weight Watchers meetings or feeding me diet shakes and fat-free frozen meals that tasted about as good as you'd imagine. Her attempts at getting me to lose weight sometimes worked, and I plodded through my teen years in a constant cycle of chubby, chubbier, and fat, then back again. Of course I wanted these dieting forays to stick, too. I saw my body as an annoying roadblock that was getting in the way of the rest of my life. But, much like the Juniors clothes I attempted to squish into, nothing I tried seemed to work.

The Lane Bryant sign in front of me seemed to glisten. "Just . . . a real quick look?" I asked again as I shifted my weight from left to right, left to right—and Mom finally relented, dismissively saying that she'd wait on the bench outside the store.

But it turned out she was right. The clothes didn't fit me. Though the store did indeed carry a size fourteen, the clothes were built for a shape different from mine. The jeans had extra space beneath the waist; the dresses were roomier in the shoulders and armpits. They fit me, but didn't. I wasn't plus sized, but I wasn't regular sized, either. I was the perfect size for the oft-forgotten make-your-own-fucking-clothes demographic.

Mom seemed to be relieved that Lane Bryant did not work for her floundering daughter; which isn't to say she didn't understand my extreme frustration. She was certainly capable of being empathic, and she understood—probably more than most—the dire importance of looking good. When I left the store empty-handed and joined her on the bench, she looked at me kindly and delicately moved a strand of hair out of my face, tucking it behind my ear. "I'm sorry, sweetie," she said, meaning it. Despite her ambivalence about her kid venturing into the world of plus sizes, she wanted nothing more than for me to be happy, comfortable, and maybe a little bit more ordinary.

Thankfully, in the early and mid-1990s, wide-legged, elastic-waist palazzo pants were in style, probably because I and I alone kept up the demand. Pair them with an oversized sweater, and you've got yourself a shapeless, hidden teenage girl. But at least the clothes fit.

Despite the fact that I felt safe enough and hidden enough inside my palatial outfits, at school my eclectic clothes, wide black head-band, waist-length black hair, and thick black eyeliner made me an easy target. I looked a little like Mama Cass, which doesn't quite gel when you're trying to get through the day without being made fun of. Thus, navigating the rather brutal social scene of the average American high school was, shall we say, challenging.

But I found ways to get by. When it wasn't food that was comforting me, it was theater. I was excellent at it, a natural, and though the oddball actor kids didn't exactly welcome me with open arms, neither did they seem to care that I was fat, and they carved out a place for me—and it was there that I thrived. I entered acting competitions and won them—including the prestigious New Jersey Governor's Award for the Arts (the category was Improvisation). But it was during a performance about date rape, which we had to present in front of our whole school because it was considered "educational material," that my two very polar worlds (the freeness of theater and the confinement of class) came crashing together.

Because of my girth, and my by-now ginormous breasts, I always played the adult characters. Frequently, they were the juicier roles, and though I knew that, I longed to be the ingénue anyway. For this particular play, my role was the therapist—not exactly juicy, but a good fit for me since it required a student who looked ages older than her still-developing peers. Frustratingly, it was a small part (there are no small parts, only fat actors) and I only appeared during the last scene. I stood backstage and waited as the play unfolded, and during the second-to-last blackout, I took my place on the chair left stage center.

The lights came back on, and within ten seconds, I was assaulted by the roar of hundreds of unseen voices. It had started with just a few heckles—hisses, cackles, boos—and those instigators paved the way for more and more insults, until the auditorium was buzzing with a raucous din of uncontrollable students, my peers. I was like an elephant in a zoo—confined and confused, an easy target. I was in the spotlight, literally, and had no choice but to sit there and stare silently at my scene partner, Kara, until it became quiet enough for me to get out my first line.

In class, when I'd walk to the front of the room to get the bathroom key, I could willingly choose not to respond to the insults. But on this stage, I had no choice but to remain in character, keeping my gaze on Kara—who, after a few seconds, awkwardly looked down at her feet, refusing to bear any of the pain alongside me. Perhaps even more than the audience's sharp words being poured onto me like buckets of pig's blood (*Carrie, I have long felt your pain*), it was Kara's turning away—her subtle, unstated, "I don't know you"—that got to me the most, branding my heart with the reality that I was on that stage and in this world all by myself.

When the teachers and principal finally shushed the students, I delivered my first line, and the heckling picked up again. I managed to finish the scene, but not unscathed. My classmates had taken my one diamond—my acting, my make-believe world where I could be anyone—and shattered it, and shattered me. I walked offstage, shaken and weeping, with one comforting thought in the back of my head: "Tonight, I will go to Burger King."

Food, especially fast food, had not faded in its ability to comfort me as I stumbled through adolescence. If anything, I loved it more and more each year that passed. Double cheeseburgers were now the name of the game—providing me with the steadiness and solace that I coveted. They were always there, always the same. Of course, there was a darker side to this relationship. Perhaps not surprisingly, the more of them I ate, the more of them I craved. They satisfied me, until they didn't. They assuaged my angst, until the absence of them added to that angst. Such is the definition of an addictive relationship—not that I thought of it that way then. But I wasn't stupid, and I knew that I was somehow in the middle of a vicious cycle of eating crappy food and then feeling crappy about my body.

Still, my love was too strong to resist. By the time I got a car— an enchanting 1986 Toyota Camry that I called "Henry," which only accelerated (barely) if you stepped full-force on the gas pedal—there was no longer an obstacle between me and eating a second (or sometimes third) dinner. The fact that I was petrified of driving on highways was not a problem—just down the road was a strip mall with everything I could ever need: a grocery store, a Chinese place, a pizza joint, a brand-new shiny Taco Bell, and, of course, my first and still greatest love, Burger King. A tub of chocolate icing from Foodtown was the perfect appetizer to a dinner of two cheeseburgers, extra-large fries, and a vanilla milk shake. The blessed drive-through was like icing on the cake (or the pie, as it were—since the apple pie at Burger King was always an option to go with the shake). I would sit in the hidden part of the parking lot, blasting my Patti LuPone cassette and eating my dinner at record speed.

It was how I imagined heaven. I scoffed to myself when I thought of those kids who—like me—wanted a buzz, but wasted their money and their brain cells on drugs, when they could have this much better, cheaper, legal, and more functional high. Who needed marijuana when you could have the perfect, orgasmic combination of fatty, sweet, and salty that made French fries with ketchup so succulent?

While my teenage journals were full of incredibly tormented poetry that made Sylvia Plath sound like Dr. Seuss, what I really should have been doing was writing love sonnets to my cheeseburger. Nestled behind the protective shield of Henry (whom I perhaps anthropomorphized a bit too readily), I finally felt *genuine*. I took a bite of my burger and I was myself. There was no other place in my life—not even in theater, not since the incident with the heckling—where I was safer, where I was calmer. I sipped my shake and, in my head, I had already escaped to New York City—where I knew I would live one day, though I wasn't entirely sure whether I wanted to be there so that I could achieve anonymity or fame.

As I took a break from my burger and dug deeper into my tub

of icing, my hopes and fears arm wrestled in my head, both certain they were destined to win: I will be incredibly famous. (I will be amazingly fat.) I will star on Broadway. (I will be ugly.) I will be rich. (I will be a failure.) I will be legendary. (I will be forgotten.) I will be loved. (I will be loathed.)

I found that the faster I ate, the more rapidly my desires pushed my fears away, and the faster the image of Margaret and my other bullying classmates faded. So I picked up the pace and sprinted to the finish, licking my fingers to make sure no morsel would go undigested. I ate until I didn't remember that I was a reject, or at least until I didn't care.

My stomach and heart swelled with satisfaction, and I felt full of life. The irony, of course, is that it was death I was full of—but I didn't see it that way for years. At the time, I was simply awaiting the cosmic high I received from the buttery bun, the smoky patty, the smooth shake that tingled as it slid down my throat into my soul and grounded me at my foundation.

One place where I was already full was my bosom. I had developed fast and early—getting my period for the first time at just nine years old. I had been visiting my father when it first arrived, and I thought that perhaps I hadn't wiped my butt properly (they never tell you that one's first period is usually a gross brown). When I showed my mother later that day, while I was complaining of a stomachache, she gave me a maxipad and called my grandmother, who, perhaps overcompensating for her distress that her nine-year-old granddaughter was, at least physically, entering womanhood, inexplicably gushed and kvelled, shouting "Mazel tov!" over and over. And then my mother proceeded to explain to me what a period was. I was only in fourth grade at the time, and sex ed didn't start until fifth.

Though girls are menstruating earlier and earlier every year, nine was still highly unusual. And so after my first cycle, Mom took me to my pediatrician, Dr. Lorn, to see if everything was okay. Dr. Lorn, a short, middle-aged man with a Hitler mustache, asked Mom to leave the room and then told me to undress. Though I was only nine, I was already very protective of my body and knew all too well that the parts that I should be shy about—maybe even ashamed of?—were the parts I hid with clothes. Dr. Lorn became impatient with me as I simply stared at him, failing to answer, until I finally started to slowly take my clothes off. He told me to lie back on the table—so I did. He told me to inch my butt down to the bottom of the table—so I did. And then he told me to spread my legs so that he could take a look.

Instead, I decided to get lost inside my brain.

I pictured my Saturday morning cartoons, which I had watched just a few hours earlier, and I lingered on a mental image of *Alvin and the Chipmunks*. Alvin was so mischievous! Always getting into trouble! But I thought Theodore was by far the cutest.

"Jasmin, do as I say," Dr. Lorn ordered—not raising his voice exactly, but remaining firm in his request.

Was this normal? I actually still don't know the answer to that. Plenty of pediatricians examine their little patients naked. So why did this feel so fucking horrible?

My body was my body. I knew that I had control over it or, at least, that I was supposed to. I didn't let my brother pinch me just as I didn't let my stepfather tickle me, so why would I let Dr. Lorn force my knees apart so that he could inspect a part of me that nobody had ever seen that way—not even me?

And yet he did anyway. When I lay down on my back, completely naked, refusing to "let my knees fall to the sides," he pried them apart for me. He pushed my legs open and started to touch my vulva. He got close and looked at me for far too many seconds, or minutes, or eons—I'm not sure which.

For years afterward, on bad days—when I would grab my stomach by the fistful and scream, when people on the street would call me a cow, when I would be so tired of living that I would become physically numb, and the only recourse would be to dig my sharp nails into my wrists and arms just so that I would feel *something*—that memory would intrusively creep back in without my consent, and once again, Dr. Lorn was right there looking.

As I lay there on my back, I was absolutely, completely mortified. I knew that my mother was just outside the room waiting, and yet even though I desperately wanted or needed an out, the very last thing in the world I wanted was for Mom to see me that way. And so I held my breath and let Dr. Lorn examine me in this incredibly inappropriate way that decades later still perplexes and infuriates me.

When he was done, I noticed a very tiny but undoubted half smile on his face. Dr. Lorn told me to put on my underwear, and that I obeyed. My mother was invited back in the room, and Dr. Lorn promptly told her that it was impossible for me to have gotten my period yet. My mother protested—she had seen it herself, for five days as I menstruated and she patiently worked with me as I figured out how to use and dispose of a maxipad. Dr. Lorn reiterated, "Not possible," then explained to my mother precisely how much pubic hair I had, the still-soft texture of it, and that I was only at the very beginning of puberty.

I sat motionless, looking down, in a purple undershirt and pink underwear. In a moment of silence, as my mother was busy shaking her head because she still didn't accept what he had to say, I meekly asked if I could please change back.

Dr. Lorn shocked both Mom and me when he guffawed. "No, honey, you can't change back." He had thought I was asking if my body could change back. Could my "soft pubic hair" ungrow and could my "breast buds" pop back into my chest?

Mom was finally at the end of her rope at that point. I could hear it in her voice. "She means, can she change back into her *clothes*, Dr. Lorn?" Mom's eyes were slightly squinted, her lips pursed.

When we got into the car a few minutes later, I sobbed and drooled. I told my mother that I would never go back to see him. She asked me what had happened, but I refused to speak—I just wept, as Mom rubbed tiny circles on my back and whispered, "Shhhh . . ."

Puberty was not off to a great start. It was fast and maniacal and took hold of my body with determination and gripped my heart with confusion.

Although my breasts had already begun budding at the time I got my first period, I could never have imagined what was about to happen to them. By the time I was thirteen, they had exploded into a nightmarish triple D. There was no hiding them, but I did my level best, insisting on wearing two "minimizer bras" at a time, in an effort to keep "Mork and Mindy"—my tongue-in-cheek names for my new constant companions—at bay as much as possible.

Then, one day in eighth grade, hope appeared on the horizon. I had gotten a teen fashion magazine and, thumbing through it right before English class, I found a story about a high school student who had had a breast reduction. My heart leapt. *You can make them smaller?!* I had to put the magazine away when class started, but later, after I turned in my quiz—which I rushed through willy-nilly—I took the magazine back out, desperate to read about what this new-to-me surgery entailed.

Of course, English class was probably a poor time to read about something so provocative, with my taunting classmates sitting around me in each direction. When Bob, who sat behind me, caught a momentary glimpse of the words "breast" and "surgery" in the article, he of course deduced that I was planning breast augmentation surgery—which was completely hilarious to him and the other kids he quickly whispered to. "Your tits aren't big enough already, Jazz?" they taunted.

But even their jabs couldn't repress my excitement at ridding myself of my mammary burden. My breasts were most certainly big enough, and then some. My mother—a modest 32B—was just as perplexed as I was by my overly endowed chest. It was a source of concern to both her and Grandma, who were pained by my enormous breasts and witnessed how they kept me separated from the kids at school in yet another dimension.

By the time I was in ninth grade, men started noticing, too. On one particularly warm September afternoon, I decided to walk home from school instead of grabbing a ride with one of my classmates who lived nearby. I was wearing a sleeveless, form-fitting denim shirt with a collar, and—naturally—black palazzo pants. There was, as always, a quarter-sized space in between the second and third buttons of my shirt. Nothing ever seemed to fit. My army jacket was tied around my waist, my backpack draped on one shoulder, and my thick hair pulled back into a messy ponytail. I chewed my Bazooka and hummed show tunes to myself as I walked the mile and a half home.

As soon as the royal blue Honda on the usually busy Grove Avenue started to slow down, I somehow knew there was going to be trouble. I looked around and, alarmingly, there was nobody in sight—nor any other vehicles anywhere to be seen. The Honda was going the same pace as me now, and so I sped up, as if that would make a difference. The unkempt, middle-aged man driving it rolled down his window and tipped his giant sunglasses a bit so that he could look over them. "Hey, sweetheart," he said. I ignored him, spotting out of the corner of my eye some woods that I knew reached to the other side of my house, popping out near my backyard. "Nice tits for a little girl," he continued, as I bolted for the woods. He promptly drove off, but in retrospect, I'm not sure if running into an even more desolate place as I was being ogled by a perverted, older man was my smartest maneuver of all time.

And they just kept growing.

By tenth grade, angry red stretch marks lined the sides of my breasts, welt-sized proclamations that Mork and Mindy didn't want to be there any more than I wanted them. By the end of each day, my entire back ached, and my shoulders had pink, bra-strap-shaped creases that were tender to the touch. The skin under them never had space to breathe, and so I would apply baby powder twice a day in hopes that it would help the chafing, though nothing really seemed to. The skin there was raw and warm, frequently dotted with painful blisters.

Though I hated them, there was no escaping them, ever. Morning, noon, and night, there they were. Nevertheless, I did my best to find ways to get along with them. One way was by finding mentors and idols who had a similar affliction but didn't let it hinder them. I wanted real evidence and validation that one day, when I got out of this small-minded, horrid place and time, I could maybe, perhaps, learn to be comfortable in my own skin. Did this possibility exist?

It existed in Bette. Gradually, as I got older and my chest got bigger, my bedroom transformed from a pink, doll-laden wonderland to a shrine dedicated to my favorite star, Bette Midler. I was truly infatuated—obsessed, really—with Bette. In addition to being in complete awe of her talent, and wanting nothing more than to grow up to be just like her, I was fascinated by the way she used her own big breasts to her benefit. As I worked my way through memorizing the lyrics and melodies to my entire collection of albums, movies, and bootleg VHS tapes of old shows, I found myself particularly infatuated with her Sophie Tucker impressions—in which she repeatedly joked about her breasts in such a way that *she was in on the joke*, which was something I longed to be. ("I was in bed with my boyfriend Herbie, and he said, 'Soph, you've got a flat chest,' and I said, 'Herbie, get off my back!'")

And then I watched in awe as Bette's boobs became the stars of the show when she flamboyantly performed the song "Otto Titsling" in the movie *Beaches*—about the fictional character who invented the brassiere—which was precisely when I knew that I was her biggest and best fan, and always would be. (Her rendition of "Pretty Legs and Great Big Knockers" from her concert, *Art or Bust*—which I owned on VHS—pretty much gave me a seizure.)

Still, being a chubby teenager with enormous breasts is harder to pull off than being a movie star with them, and real-life New Jersey was not kind to me—or to Mork and Mindy. My TM was distressed, and her concern grew as I did. When I passed her bedroom one night and heard her on the phone chatting with

Grandma, I detected that her voice was notably soft—proving to me two things: (1) she was trying to be secretive, and (2) it was my mission to find out what she was talking about.

"She's so matronly," I heard her say as I pressed my ear to her door in the spot that I had previously determined (with loads of practice) was the easiest to hear through. "I really don't know how to handle it," Mom continued. "She's much bigger than the other kids at school—which they never stop reminding her of. And she's so unhappy all the time."

Admittedly, everything Mom said was entirely accurate, but hearing my mother, size four her whole adult life, call me "matronly" absolutely stung anyway. It wasn't that I didn't sense her discomfort about my body size, and it also wasn't as if she'd really said anything wrong or insensitive. But "matronly" was just not a word that I wanted associated with me, regardless of how true it was. I wanted to rip my flesh off my skeleton and put it through a shredder.

It was my TM who first brought up the possibility of my having a breast reduction. I was sitting in the kitchen eating a bowl of chocolate ice cream with Cool Whip and gummy bears when she came in and sat down beside me. *For the Boys*, starring, of course, Bette Midler, was playing (once again) on the nearby VCR. "What?" I asked curtly, with a mouthful of ice cream, and a chocolaty chin.

"Jazz . . ." She momentarily hesitated, eyeballing my heaping bowl. "I thought maybe you would want to consider having a breast reduction."

My spoon fell into my bowl. Bette's rendition of "In My Life" faded into the background, and immediately I was as present as I could be—this was suddenly *my life.*

I thought back to the article I had read a few years prior, about the teenager who'd had a reduction. It had never occurred to me that getting one was an actual real possibility—I thought it was just for people in magazines. Even though Mom's suggestion stunned me, it occurred to me that I should have seen it coming. She had long been concerned about my "situation" and was craving a solution almost as much as I was. And since putting my body through a shredder was off the table, at sixteen, during the summer between my junior and senior year of high school, I went through with the surgery.

It turned out that getting that breast reduction was the best thing I could have possibly done. It was my first foray into understanding how relatively simple it was to permanently alter my body and establish my ownership of it. In the years to come, I would continue to gain and lose weight over and over, and then, eventually, lose nearly one hundred pounds and keep it off. I would get one tattoo, then another, and end up with more tattooed body parts than not. I would pierce things and shave my head. I would do whatever I could to alter, hide from, and, ultimately, reclaim and liberate my body.

Perhaps getting a breast reduction was my first taste of that reclamation. Because when I returned to school in the fall, as a senior, things were very different. I busied my brain solidifying my plans to become a legendary actress—a plan that required quite a lot of thought and daydreaming. I had one foot out of the door already— *I desperately wanted out.* I joined Future Teachers of America for the sole purpose of missing a day of school each week so that I could student teach, and I applied for—and received—the privilege some seniors get of "early release," making my school day a lot shorter than that of most kids. During the few times when I was actually in school, I would simply cut—whenever and however possible.

As far as I was concerned, I was already out of high school. I was already independent. In my head, I already had my own apartment in the city, and—just like Bette—the world already understood and accepted me. In this fantasy, my body became a nonentity and people saw me for my talent instead. In my daydreams, I got parts, and I got boyfriends. In my head, I was already somebody.

During my senior year, it wasn't just my fantasy world that changed. The real world changed, too. My body was radically different and it was difficult for even me to recognize myself in the mirror. Motivated by my smaller-seeming frame, and physically weakened during recovery from the surgery, I had managed to shed a few pounds that summer, too. Just having a smaller chest gave the impression that I had lost weight, and my relatively minor weight loss on top of that made me look like a different girl altogether. My classmates simply stared, stymied by how different I looked, unable to pinpoint the exact cause of it.

And while my peers didn't exactly start to be nice, their attitude was one of the things that changed that year. When that same Margaret from my history class suddenly and vehemently changed her go-to insult to me from "Fat-Ass" to "Ho," I stood a little straighter and smiled, just a bit, to myself: I knew that it meant I was a tad less of a pariah than before. "Ho," after all, was a way more desirable gibe. Finally, I was getting places.

I remember that afternoon I was called a "ho": It was the first time I was degraded in a way that had nothing whatsoever to do with my size. That same night, I memorialized what I felt was a huge accomplishment with a celebratory milk shake and a tub of icing. The future was looking sweet.

FOUR

—

you couldn't ignore a girl in green overalls if you tried

When I went off to college, I gained back all the weight I had lost the previous year. Hardly a unique story for college freshmen, who often taste independence for the first time just as enthusiastically as they taste late-night diner food and cheap beer. Even Mork and Mindy reappeared for their "Where Are They Now?" special, growing back to some extent, as the rest of me filled out to bigger than I had been before.

In an act of complete ludicrousness, my TM would not allow me to go to college in New York City, feeling it was "too dangerous." So she sent me an hour and a half in the opposite direction instead, to Philadelphia (which, for what it's worth, has way higher crime rates than New York). When I received a substantial scholarship to study for my bachelor of fine arts in acting at the University of the Arts, the choice was really made for me anyway.

I remember standing on Anna Lane retrieving the mail from our wooden, house-shaped mailbox at the end of the driveway when I got the notice of my scholarship. I stood there and opened the envelope: *Dear Miss Singer: We are pleased to inform you that* . . . I let out a little scream, no doubt startling everyone on my sleepy street, then decided to sit on the curb until Mom got home so that I could tell her the news immediately. When I spotted her Saturn coming down Anna Lane, I ran toward it as if the house was on fire, which, when she saw me, she thought it was. "I got in! I got a scholarship! I got in! I got a scholarship!" I kept yelling, until she was able to decipher my slurred, screeching words.

The school was, ironically, my mother's alma mater—back when it had been Philadelphia College of Art—and the theater program there was selective, small, and well established. So even though I was disappointed by New York City being off the table, I was sufficiently wooed by the respectable theater education I'd get and flattered by my scholarship. Plus, I craved living in a big city with every ounce of longing I had—anything to get me out of Edison!—and I saw the move as a huge step in the right direction, even if that right direction was taking me in the opposite one from the city I dreamed of, the city shimmering with Broadway lights, the city where I'd eventually land.

Finally, a fresh start! I could leave my bullied days behind me, trade in my despair for hope and my burger for a cheesesteak.

Plus, hell had apparently frozen over, because I had a boyfriend. A real-life, blond-haired and blue-eyed, crazy-about-me boyfriend. Timmy was twenty-five to my seventeen; worldly to my still-sheltered; rough-around-the-edges to my pseudo-sophisticated; a daredevil to my play-by-the-rules. And yet we went together as perfectly as a Boston cream donut goes with a Dunkin' Donuts Coffee Coolatta (my drink of choice, which Timmy always picked up for me on his way to our outings). We met in summer stock (that's a repertory company that performs plays only in June, July, and August) during the summer after high school and fell madly, unabashedly in love. He was tasked with the nightly duty of helping me with a quick costume change, and then he'd bring my worn jeans back to the dressing room. Little did I know then that he was pretty much having a relationship with those jeans, and plotting how to move on past denim and make his first move with me. Timmy could have been a star on a soap opera. He was stereotypically gorgeous in a "surfer dude" kind of way, and the two of us made an odd-looking, but deeply devoted pair.

Despite his good looks, Timmy didn't have much more dating experience than I did, and so we both threw ourselves into our relationship with urgency, each of us trying to make up for lost time by loving harder. Though Timmy was stunning, he, too, had felt like an outcast his whole life. His mother had been unwell and severely mentally imbalanced, and he had diverted his attention away from his problems at home by diving into the world of motocross racing. For his whole life, the worlds of motocross and grunge had defined him, leaving his love life on the sidelines—until I came around and, for the first time, he opened his heart.

The summer in between my senior year of high school and my freshman year of college—the Summer of Timmy—was the most magical of my life, full of self-expression and adventure, realized lust, deeply felt emotion, and awkward but sweet lovemaking. All this was the exact opposite of what my school days had been like, and I basked in my newfound freedom with a profound and almost jarring ecstasy.

Seeing myself through the eyes of a doting boyfriend who

wanted to worship my body—the same body that had been the target of ridicule by my loathsome classmates mere *weeks* prior—I began to wonder if my dark days were behind me. I had sincere hope that my new life in Philadelphia would bring with it a redefinition that I desperately craved—one that Timmy jump-started when he looked at me and called me beautiful.

Timmy moved me into my Center City apartment at the end of August, following my final performance as an oddly cast Honey in *Who's Afraid of Virginia Woolf?* which costarred *Welcome Back, Kotter*'s Ron Palillo—a B-level celebrity with whom I was enamored and starstruck. Surely my close proximity to this level of fame—*He knew John Travolta! The boy in the bubble!*—meant that I, myself, would soon be discovered. Timmy and I drove over the Delaware River quietly singing Tori Amos's version of "Smells Like Teen Spirit," and I gawked with hesitant but exhilarating excitement as the skyline of my brand-new city got bigger. Hours later, I kissed Timmy good-bye for twenty minutes, wanting him to stay but needing him to go. It was time for me to start again.

I entered my first Acting Studio class in college wearing fluorescent green satin overalls. "Be brave," I had whispered to myself that morning, as I stared in the mirror at my reflection, pleased that I was beginning to strongly resemble a young, if larger, Liza Minnelli—a resemblance that I did my best to enhance with my short, jet-black hair and heavy, dramatic bangs, as well as the requisite black eyeliner that extended out onto my temples. I was as gung ho on making an impression as I was on making a name for myself, and that kind of prominence—I was sure—began with an eclectic wardrobe. So my choice to wear green satin overalls was indeed premeditated. You couldn't ignore a girl in green overalls if you tried.

My new peers didn't ignore me, but they didn't care all that much, either. That was the first thing I noticed about the students who made up my conservatory theater program—being offbeat was not the thing that got you noticed, it was the thing that got you in the door. My theater program was, in essence, a collection of wildly talented small-town weirdos, suburban outcasts, and red-headed stepchildren. We were the ones who just didn't fit: the driven ones, the fat ones, the gay ones, the activist ones, and, yes, the bullied ones. And, finally, we were able to celebrate ourselves and each other—beginning with the common denominator of not fitting into the suburban hells most of us had come from. My freshman year of college was like a slightly glorified, older, gayer version of *Fame*. We might as well have danced on cars, because we were absolutely going to live forever. Each and every one of us was going to be a star—that we knew. We had the talent and ambition to make it happen.

But first, we had to regulate our antidepressants.

Put a bunch of talented rejects in a room, and you can bet your Broadway bootleg that the vast majority are keeping the pharmaceutical industry very comfortable by consuming their fair share of mood stabilizers. That was true in spades with my Acting Studio class, a tiny and passionate group of young actors who took our craft as seriously as we took our black eyeliner. (It wasn't just me who loaded it on. Others, apparently, were also under the impression that the more eyeliner you wore, the less you needed to explain yourself. I still think there's some truth in that.) In fact, if you were depressed—or, even better, bipolar!—you were given an extra level of respect and secretly expected to perform better monologues.

It will perhaps not come as a surprise at this point that depression had been no stranger to me throughout my teen years. It frequently enveloped me, especially when all the taunting made it seem like too much for me to get through my high school classes. I would use my hair as a curtain and my sleeves as a tissue. My obsession with Sylvia Plath certainly didn't help matters much. It seemed I was a classic teenage sucker for angst and misery.

But then, after my sleeve was sufficiently soggy and my eyeliner effectively smeared, I would spiral down further into the depths of despair—traveling far beyond a momentary and justified upset. Things I normally enjoyed—like listening to music, reading novels, and writing poetry—had no meaning for me. The only thing that mattered during those times was food—my one constant, reliable source of satisfaction. Depression was no match against a row of Oreos or a box of Cheez-Its.

When I was fourteen, my TM had insisted on getting me into therapy—my intense moods and darkness were frightening to her. I would write morbid poetry on a daily basis, mostly about broken romances that I'd never experienced except in my head. No doubt tragic lost love seemed like a more noble and exciting excuse for my broken heart than being ostracized by everyone at school. When my therapist suggested I consider going on Prozac—a relatively new drug that still carried with it a social stigma (almost as much as wearing plus-size clothing)—Mom adamantly refused. What would it mean to have a young daughter who needed a pill to get happy? What kind of failure would that make her?

So, during my freshman year of college, when it became clear that I was the lone kid in my Acting Studio class who wasn't on the happy pill, I began to wonder if I should be.

Still, being a person of somewhat dramatic emotional range, I've never found misery incompatible with ecstasy, and I was indeed euphoric to be away at college. During those first few months, I drank Philadelphia up until it was dry. My eager classmates and I would spend our evenings on South Street getting plastered at one of the many bars that didn't check IDs (and I'd spend the next morning swearing that I'd never drink again—until that night or the following, when I would do it all over again). And there was theater in my life, even if, for the moment, it was only tangentially. I got a job selling programs for a production of *The Phantom of the Opera*, and I became fast friends with the offbeat, bohemian crew. My wardrobe became funkier and my eyeliner heavier. I dove into my new grown-up life with a fanaticism that fulfilled and petrified me.

Not surprisingly to either of us, weeks into the semester I broke Timmy's heart by telling him that I needed to focus on my life in Philly now. "I think we should break up," I said calmly, impressed by my own detachment as he wept copiously onto my pink faux fur jacket.

As is typical for so many floundering eighteen-year-olds (and I was no exception), my breakup was not only self-centered, but seriously overstated. But while I may have drawn the curtain on act 1, Timmy's and my future together was still waiting in the wings, ready to be resuscitated and rediscovered. Our lives and hearts would be intertwined for years. In fact, even when it really was over many years later, the role that he played as my first love—the one who loved me back, even when I felt entirely unlovable—would shape me forever and would heal so many of the wounds that were still left from high school.

But I didn't have time to think about that then. The months that passed between graduating from high school and settling into my new college life had been fierce and frenetic. Between summer stock and my summer of love, moving to a new city and meeting all new peers, I could barely come up for air. I maniacally, but somewhat unconsciously, moved through my days, charged by the dazzling (and sometimes blinding) lights around me.

When my life in Philly began to settle down, I became abundantly aware that lying beneath all that constant activity was, still, depression. It became an unwanted but unshakable companion, in the same way my stomach was. The awareness of my significant size and my equally significant depression followed me around my room, my town, my life—never letting me forget they were there, that they were running the show.

Once the initial adrenaline of my new life had worn off, I realized that the dark shadow had been there all along, lurking nearby, waiting for a moment of silence to make itself known. My depression dwelled in the corner of my small apartment along with the life-sized James Dean cardboard cutout that I propped up near the window to trick robbers into thinking I wasn't home alone.

And my round stomach with pink stretch marks came with me to voice class, where it bounced up and down, out and in, left and right, as I learned how to properly inhale and exhale, the actor way. (Apparently, actors breathe differently than other mortals.)

My depression sat quietly while I'd eat a cheeseburger at Johnny Rockets with my friends, only feeling safe enough to fully emerge when I got home a few hours later.

During that same outing to Johnny Rockets, my stomach would spread out on my lap like a small child, giddy because I was feeding it.

Then, late at night when I'd sit cross-legged on my living room floor wearing my favorite flannel pajamas with red kissy lips all over them, my depression would encase me like thick molasses and I would barely be able to move. So I'd go in slow motion, always aware of the extreme effort it took to get from my bed to my bathroom, my bathroom to my living room, my living room to my life. The syrup would seep its way into my ears, and when people spoke to me, they sounded distant.

I finally gathered enough gumption to seek out a new therapist. One of my motivations came from my peers, who convinced me that digging deep was key to unleashing the burgeoning Tony winner inside me. And so I gathered weeks' worth of fantasies about how much deeper an actor I'd be once I found a good shrink to help me parse out my lingering sadness. Even more importantly, I was tired of constantly being miserable.

Even among the outcast theater kids—the ones who, like me, traded in any chance of making money for the infinitely small possibility of making it as an actor—I was still a bit of a loner. I was a particular brand of "weird" that didn't sit well even among the weirdos.

The problem was, I began to realize, that my status as an outcast wasn't rooted only in the fact that I was fat. It was becoming apparent that I was simply *too much*. I was too needy, too clingy, too desperate. I was too quick to want to perform my monologue first in front of the class, too exuberant when asked to provide feedback for the other kids, too demanding of my teachers' time. It seemed I took up too much space wherever I went, not just physically, and that naturally put the others off. At the end of the day, in the quiet solitude of my tiny apartment in Center City, I felt the flip side of that "too much"—the screaming silence that ate away at me until I ate away at my feelings; the lingering lone-liness that lessened only when I found a friend in food.

Even though college gave me the independence I craved in spades, I still floated through my days with an overarching feeling of isolation, the manifestation of which was my ever-expanding body.

I needed a shrink.

When I walked in the door of my new therapist's office on Second Street just off South, and came face-to-face with Dr. Smith, I suddenly felt queasy—and it was not the aftereffect of the ice cream cone and candy bar I had anxiously devoured on the way there. The last thing I expected, and the last thing I wanted in my psychiatrist, was for her to be obese. And yet, that was exactly what she was.

Does admitting that make me a bad person? I'm not sure. But I do know that it had been a near lifetime of body and weight issues that had brought me to her in the first place, and just as an alcoholic seeking treatment would not want to smell brandy on his therapist's breath, I immediately felt I could not possibly con-fide in a therapist who was 150 pounds overweight.

Yet there I was, and I felt I had to see it through. I would stick it out, though I would never trust her. Even though I feel ashamed to admit this, I would always judge her, even more harshly than I judged myself.

My new shrink put out her hand. "I'm Dr. Smith," she said, with a smile in her eyes. I stared at her for a beat. She had silky, dark brown hair pulled back into a bun and wore a khaki-colored dress that stopped at midcalf. On her shoulders, she had draped a bright shawl. I wondered if Dr. Smith shopped at Lane Bryant. I wondered if she was ashamed of it.

Finally I shook her hand back. "Hi," was all she got out of me. "Let's sit down," she said, and we did.

I continued to be bullied, no longer by classmates, but instead by strangers—mainly men—whose behavior ranged from staring at my still very substantial rack and whispering, "God bless you," all the way to calling me names like "Fat Fuck."

When I wasn't busy with classes or gallivanting to South Street with my friends (somehow it never occurred to me or anyone else that all that drinking could have been contributing to my depression), I would take the New Jersey Transit train two hours north to New York. Though I had learned to appreciate the quaint, cobblestone pathways in Philadelphia, the rebellious spirit and raciness of South Street, and the subversive theater and dance scene there, it was still the Big Apple that I dreamed of. And so on weekends I would travel there and simply walk around aimlessly, for hours on end—or perhaps I'd hang out in the busy and bright theater district and sneak into the second half of a Broadway play during intermission—before turning around and heading back to Philadelphia, where my life and my dessert were waiting.

During one such sojourn in New York, I was crossing Fourteenth Street, humming "At the Ballet" from *A Chorus Line* and snacking on peanut M&M's, when I caught a glimpse of a man walking toward me, eyes squinting, just staring. I suspected what was about to happen—I was used to it. I quickly stuffed the M&M's in my coat pocket and made a mental note of where I was in the song so that I could pick it up again later. The man put his hands in his pockets. I looked down, kept walking. He stopped directly in front of me. There were people everywhere, but they didn't take note. I was on my own. "Fat slob," he said, an inch from my face. "Fat whore," he continued as I passed him. I walked faster.

When I was a kid, my mother had told me to ignore them. I ignored him, grasping my M&M's for dear life—they were what was normal. He was what was evil.

I was away from him finally. But he hollered back after me. "Fat fuck!" he yelled, loud enough this time for others to hear. They had to hear him. But they still didn't look up.

It took three weeks for Dr. Smith to prescribe Prozac for me. I had stuck with seeing her, mainly because I didn't have the energy to look elsewhere, and I didn't want to explain to my TM why I wanted to change therapists. Anyway, finally I had an antidepressant prescription, so perhaps my otherwise wasted time with her—during which I remained guarded and told her only what I felt I absolutely had to—had been worth it after all.

One day after class, I told the kids in my Acting Studio class about my Prozac and they nodded with sincere empathy and approval. The nine of us sat around in a circle on the floor, our legs or fingers interlaced with one another's—practically singing "Kumbaya" and having an orgy. Many of us softly cried as we each confessed why we were full of such deep despair. The stories my peers shared were harrowing. Julie's father molested her for fifteen years. Michaela was addicted to sex. Derek's father committed suicide when he was ten. It was deep shit, and hearing others' tragic real-life problems made me feel like a poseur.

In contrast to our very adult problems were our clothes—most of us, including me, were wearing pajama bottoms with T-shirts to allow for freedom of movement in class. My pajamas had spaceships all over them that day, and on the top, I wore a T-shirt from the musical *Chicago*, which I had already seen seven times—or at least seen the second half of seven times.

"What about you?" Hazel asked me. "What are your demons, Jasmin?"

"Yeah," echoed Eric. "Why the Prozac?"

I looked up from the ground, and then around at the circle of precocious eighteen-year-olds in pajamas, staring back at me.

I took a breath, not knowing how to respond. Nothing seemed big enough, valid enough, true enough. Nothing in my life could possibly make sense of the overpowering sadness that lived inside me. I had love, after all. I had privilege. I knew these things, and yet I felt like a prisoner inside myself.

Finally, I looked up at the stained ceiling and audibly exhaled. The spots on it were browner and wider than they had been the previous week. There were rumors that the building was full of asbestos, and the rumors turned out to be true, because two years later, the city mandated that the building be destroyed. But before the building was destroyed because of asbestos, I had to face my own poison. "I'm fat," I finally said. "And I fucking hate myself."

That night I baked a cake. It was the first one I ever made, and even though it came from a box (just like Mom's!), I was wickedly and irrationally proud of it. It was a chocolate layer cake with store-bought chocolate icing. When I picked up the eggs, cake mix, and icing earlier that day, I had enough good sense to buy two tubs of the icing—one of which I snacked on, in its entirety, as the cake rose in the hot oven.

And when the cake was ready, I ate it in full. And as I ate it, my heart felt full. So, with crumbs on my shirt and icing on my mouth, I whispered to Philadelphia, "The Prozac must be working."

FIVE

the perfect facade of safety

My sophomore year of college was when everything came to a head, then promptly and without warning changed the course of my life.

During the summer leading up to it, I had worked as an acting teacher at a Jewish day camp in New Jersey. There, I had tried out both my newfound ability to attract boys and my newfound sexuality, by way of an intense but short-lived relationship with a Rutgers student named Bradley. I made my choice primarily based on Bradley's talent at playing the piano and songwriting. He was also an excellent accompanist to my growing roster of show tunes.

Returning to my tiny Philadelphia apartment, where my cardboard cutout of James Dean still remained, unwavering, in the window, I fell right back into my now-familiar mix of driving ambition and deep despair. Fortunately, I still had my short-term fixes—the familiar comforts of pizza and scrambled eggs. Like my James Dean cutout, the calmness bestowed by food was reliable, always there, providing the perfect facade of safety.

I was no longer seeing Dr. Smith. I finally got fed up with her accusation, leveled at me more than once, that I was high on pot during our sessions. I wasn't. Though I laughed it off at the time, looking back I can see why she may have come to that conclusion. The truth is, she didn't trust me, and she had every right not to. I was guarded with her, never able to get past her obesity for long enough to give her a glimpse into the reasons why I ate to excess, or the reasons why despair was taking over my life.

Anyway, the main reason I had been seeing her was for the meds, though I don't actually think that the Prozac did much for my sadness (nor did it make me a better actor). In fact, an argument could be made that the extra-cheese pizza I ate every day, or (if I was feeling fancy) the cheese omelets, did a better job at keeping my depression at bay. But that was the thing: Neither the meds nor the food nor Dr. Smith helped me look more closely at the systemic reason behind why I was stuck in a hateful cycle of overeating and depression, depression and overeating, overeating and depression, and on and on. More importantly, not only did they fail to help me understand it, but they didn't help me get out of it. Gradually the depression became even more consuming than before, and I spiraled deeper and deeper.

At some point, others began to notice that I was slogging through my days. I dragged my feet, perpetually arrived a few minutes late to class, and stopped volunteering to go first (or at all). When my academic adviser, who was also one of my professors, asked me what the story was, I responded that it wasn't that I wanted to die, but that I didn't want to live, either. That obviously raised a red flag with him, and the school soon bundled me off for more sophisticated professional intervention. Thus began a new course of treatment with a group of doctors at the nearby teaching hospital. It was, in retrospect, one of the worst disasters of my life.

The hospital was only a few blocks from where I lived, yet it seemed an entire world away from the colorful land of theater arts that had defined my Philadelphia existence. The building was bright white, sterile, and lacking the charming nooks and crannies (and, presumably, asbestos) that made UArts bustle with such distinct character. I was evaluated by a young medical student whose crisp white lab coat was too large for his tiny body. He asked me some standard questions, then shuffled me to the next doctor, who asked me more questions and wrote out a scrip for an extremely heavy dose of a mood stabilizer that stabilized little more than my lack of self-worth.

Adolescent angst is a pretty scary place. The pharmaceutical industry, which claims to make it easier to navigate, is too often making it worse with medications that are unnecessary at best and addictive and damaging at worst. I'm certainly not saying that prescription medicine is never helpful, but too often the proposed solution for every misery is to simply pop a pill. And while I initially craved a pill to find validation for my feelings (anything for a quick fix), like so many others, I quickly saw the dark side of that supposed validation. Once I traveled down the well-worn path of mood-stabilizing medication, there was no stopping—until I had no other choice but to stop everything.

I don't actually remember a whole lot of details about what came next, but I do recall with a haunting clarity that I was misdiagnosed as bipolar and improperly medicated. The combination of the wrong meds and crippling self-hatred caused me to basically cease functioning almost altogether. I woke up in the mornings feeling like I was under water, my limbs like thick and soggy logs that I could hardly maneuver. I started to fall asleep in class, and when my friends invited me to South Street for a foray to Johnny Rockets, I opted instead to crawl into my unmade bed with my weeks-old sheets. My head ached and my heart felt numb.

One day, during an early morning ballet class that I had forced myself to attend, vaguely proud that I had arrived to the barre only a few minutes late for the warm-up, I went blank. I just stood there as the people around me did the warm-up routine: bending over, bending back, and again. My intention was there: "Plié," I whispered to myself, as my soggy, heavy limbs dangled at my sides. But I simply could not move—my multiple medications were making me a zombie.

And so I left college.

Off I went back to New Jersey to stay with my mother and Wayne. Mom was determined to get me past my zombie state, and so after making sure I was under the care of a much more competent psychologist, she encouraged me to audition for a children's play, in which, thankfully, I was cast. This was a role that paid actual money (at least enough for a coffee) and made me feel like a working actor. When people asked why I was suddenly back home, I went with the bogus story that I had left school in order to be in this play, rather than the truth: that I had left school because after years of self-medicating depression with cheese, I had been wrongly medicated with equally legal, but much more powerful, pharmaceuticals. As a result, I had suffered a mental breakdown. I'm sure that they preferred hearing the fake story. I certainly preferred telling it.

Only a week after returning to Mom's from Philadelphia, I met Richard. There have been so many times throughout the past fifteen years that I have wished I could just pluck him out of my story, but I can't. He's embedded in it as permanently and as deeply as the scars and stretch marks all over my body.

My friend Vera had made it her personal mission to cheer me up, and so she insisted that we take an afternoon trip over to the college town of New Brunswick, New Jersey, where, coincidentally, my brother, Jeremy, was living at the time. Jeremy was a recent college grad who spent his days canvassing with the environmental group NJPIRG.

Though I hadn't spent much time there, New Brunswick and I went way back: I had been born there nineteen years earlier and I'd also had my breast reduction there. So, when I made eye contact with an older man who worked at a record store that Vera and I popped into, I thought surely the third great thing to happen to me here would be meeting my soul mate. That was the way I thought—always looking for the quick fix. Perhaps meeting a romantic partner would solve all my problems, make life right again. At the very least, a little harmless flirtation and mutual desire would create a welcome distraction from living, once again, on Anna Lane and under the watchful eye of my TM.

Richard had a shaved head and pronounced jaw and wore faded jeans and steel-toed combat boots. He was older—that was clear—though it wasn't until our first date (of two total) that I found out that he was thirty-five. I pretended that it didn't faze me, figuring that if I was seemingly unflappable about it I would seem more mature.

In spite of my sojourn with Timmy, and my quick fling with Bradley, it was still highly unusual for men to give me attention of the positive variety, and yet Richard was clearly fixated on me, repeatedly asking me the kinds of things that men ask women they are trying to pick up, but which I'd never heard from anyone before: Could he help me find a particular album? Did I go to Rutgers? Was I new in town? Because *surely he would have remembered me if he'd seen me before*, he said.

Vera pulled me into the classic rock section, her eyes glimmering. "See, Jazz, things are looking up for you!" She was practically giddy, and her excitement made me shyly smile. I had been a sad sack for months, and I wondered sometimes if those close to me in my life had more invested in me getting happy than I did. When Richard asked for my number, I was astonished and wondered, momentarily, if he was making fun of me.

A few days later, we met at a diner, where we both ordered cheese omelets with steak fries, then shared a scoop of lemon sorbet (in truth, I wanted my own scoop). Afterward, we sat in Richard's car (a *true* lemon) and made out like teenagers—which, in fact, I was. Richard wore circular, wire-framed eyeglasses that night (making him look more intellectual than when we'd met a few days prior), but placed them in the glove compartment during a breather from our make-out session. That was when he told me what I had always been dying to hear—that, had I been around in the 1940s, my curves would have made me a model. Bolstered by this praise, I decided to tell him that I was self-conscious about my weight. He responded by lightly grazing his hands over my shape and saying, "No, no, babe . . . you're exactly the right size . . . Who wants a skinny bitch, anyway? You're succulent."

I was hooked.

On our second date, I drove right past my brother Jeremy's place on the way to Richard's. Jeremy lived in a communal house known widely as the Purple House, for it was a bright, jewel-colored purple—and it always reeked of pot.

I did not intend to have sex with Richard that night. Though I was not a virgin, the only two men I had been with by that point had each been my boyfriend at the time, and sex was not something I simply jumped into.

Richard's housemate was home, so we mainly hung out in his room in order to have our privacy. I slowly walked around, taking in the space, stopping at carefully framed photos of his family—his sister, his mother, his nephews. "They're all cute," I said. I thought only a really good guy would have his family's photos hanging up.

We started kissing, and it was clear Richard wanted to do more. So I decided to set my first boundary of the evening. We were sitting on the side of his bed, feet on the ground. He was focused on my neck, giving me room to speak. "Hey, Richard, I don't want to have sex, okay?"

He kept going at it with my neck and finally mumbled, "Mmm-hmmm." We continued to make out, and he started to undress himself, then me, calling me luscious, gorgeous, and captivating. "You should just always be naked," he said, making me cackle, flattering and embarrassing me.

"Richard, I don't want to have sex," I reiterated a few hot minutes later, though from a smaller, further-away place. This time, he ignored me.

It was late—around midnight—and it was absolutely pouring

outside. Thunder clapped and bright bolts of lightning momentarily lit up his otherwise dark bedroom. I started to wonder where I'd sleep that night. I was growing uncomfortable, even though I also craved the attention Richard was giving me. I was caught between two polar feelings: how confined I was starting to feel with Richard all over me and how freeing it felt to be kissed and complimented.

I looked down at my body. It was dark in the room, but I could still make out the red scars on my breasts from my surgery just three years earlier, scars I had forced myself to explain to him moments earlier—and had to demystify for every other person I slept with—in a somewhat awkward way, because how do you bring something like that up in the heat of the moment?

My stomach was round, with a deep, vertical crease in the middle that made me feel I was somehow blessed with two of them. My thighs and arms were full and fleshy, and yet Richard seemed to think that my extra padding was "succulent"—so maybe it was?

Soon he was on top of me, and it became clear what was happening. I knew I needed to manage the situation, but I didn't know exactly what it was I had gotten myself into. Even in retrospect, I am perplexed by the decision making that led to my being in a thirty-five-year-old's bedroom, completely naked, proclaiming that I didn't want to have sex. It's not as though I blame myself, exactly, for the events that were about to unfold, but I was not taking care of myself—and most certainly should not have been there. I was wooed by Richard's interest in me, his obsession with my body, with my flesh. Despite the fact that I was no longer on medications, aside from an antidepressant, ever since I had been prescribed heavy doses of medication that I did not need, my body and my mind had felt detached, like two separate entities sharing space. Richard was temporarily merging those two parts of me, and I found I was thirsty for unification and affection.

"I don't want to," I said—louder and firmer than before.

"You can't do this to me, babe," he replied, also firmer.

I was silent. I shut down. It was going to happen no matter what I said, and so I asked him if he had a condom.

He did not.

I put my foot down again, as much as I could muster. "Could you please get one?" I whispered, and his shoulders stiffened up and his brow furrowed.

"God damn it, Jasmin," he said as he got off of me and out of the bed, haphazardly pulling on his clothes as he ran out of the house and down the street, in the pouring rain, to get a condom at the nearby store.

I was alone in his bed, still naked. Was this my out? I could not for the life of me figure out what to do—whether to leave, and risk running into him on my way out, or to stay and continue to pretend that things were functioning in a normal, respectful way.

My eyes welled up. I closed them and let a few tears sneak out and roll down the sides of my face, as I thought of my mother asleep in her bed—just twenty minutes away on Route 18—or my grandmother asleep in hers, a half hour in the opposite direction on the New Jersey Turnpike. The unconditional love they each had for me staggered me just then, juxtaposed with this house, this room, this moment. I felt kicked in the gut with despair. I thought of Philadelphia, just an hour and a half to the south, and wondered if my former classmates were sleeping. Or perhaps they were on South Street getting looks and getting drunk. I was, I knew, just a distant memory to them already. I didn't matter to them anymore, not nearly as much as I mattered right in that moment to Richard, who walked back into his bedroom in what seemed like just a few short minutes later—completely drenched and mildly out of breath, but carrying a small plastic black bag of condoms.

I still didn't want to have sex with him. I saw no way out.

In a last-ditch effort—and fueled by the fleeting self-respect I tapped into as I thought of how important my friends and family were to me, and perhaps how important I was to them—I tried to find a way out anyway. And so mere moments after Richard returned from the store, when he was on top of me once again, trying to find the erection he had lost, I grasped at my last shreds of self-worth and said, "Richard, I'm sorry, but I don't want to."

He ignored me, tried to fumble with the condom. It became clear that he could not get an erection with the condom.

My voice became tiny—yet it was still there, I was sure of it. And even though I barely heard myself say, "Richard, no," *I said it*—and Richard heard, too, because he hit the pillow above me with all his might and once again said—louder, this time—"God damn it, Jasmin!"

Perhaps it was a couple of hours too late, but at that moment I tried but failed to get up and out of the bed, and into my clothes and into my car, and onto the highway and back to my life—away from Richard, away from this house, away from this city where I was born and where I then worried I might also die.

But Richard pushed all his weight on me so I couldn't move. He threw the condom across the room and was suddenly hard again. "Richard, *no!*" I said—much louder this time—while he pulled my arms above my head and held me down. Then he penetrated me, harsh and defiant, detached and violent.

I whimpered, "No," for the final time.

The rain outside seemed to come down harder—the thunder rumbled again and again, building. I closed my eyes and imagined I was outside staring up at the sky, with rain falling all around me but miraculously not on me. I was immune to the water, to the weather, to the storm. In my head, I simply observed the raging rain and growling thunder in every direction—above me, around me, inside me.

Richard finished, then let go of me. And though I could have run, I lay there instead. Finally I broke my own silence by quietly reiterating the cold, hard fact. "I said no."

His back was to me, and I saw it tense up. He got up and put his jeans on, then left the room.

My arms hurt where he had held them down. I got up, too, and quickly got dressed. Richard was in the bathroom, and as I put on my second shoe, my eyes briefly stopped at the photo of his family I had gazed at earlier that evening. "You're all strangers," I whispered to them as I caught a glimpse of myself in a small hanging mirror I hadn't noticed until then. There was mascara running down my cheeks. *When did I start crying?*

I bolted down Richard's stairs and outside, but as soon as the front door slammed behind me, I realized I had forgotten my bag. I had no choice but to go back for it, since it held my car keys. When I turned around and faced the front door, I spotted a sign hanging there that I hadn't seen before: *U.S. Army: Forever Straight.*

I rang the bell, and Richard—still shirtless—opened it. I didn't make eye contact with him at first, but I tried to play it cool. "Sorry . . . I forgot my bag."

I waited there, on the porch, in the pouring rain, as Richard went to retrieve it. He came down and handed it to me, and I smiled as best I could. "Thanks," I said, nonchalantly, wondering how I was supposed to act after something like that happened.

And in a moment so brief that anyone else would have missed it, Richard's eyes finally met mine. They looked tired and sunken in, and I remember briefly wondering what ghosts he might have hidden in there. The rain poured on my head as we each stood there silently, in those final seconds together, and I tightly clutched my bag like it was my parting gift. I opened my mouth to say something inconsequential—not that I had any words left—but Richard beat me to it. "Well," was all he managed, before shutting the door and leaving me and my own ghosts, the ones I now know all too well, on his front porch.

It was two A.M. now, and the rain was unrelenting. I had no idea where to go—I could hardly go home like this—and so I drove around New Brunswick, crying openly, wondering what had just happened to me.

Stopped at a red light, I spotted out of the corner of my eye a disheveled but cute young guy on the corner, smoking a cigarette, waiting for the light to change. Even in my hysterics, I wondered why he didn't have an umbrella. I looked closer and realized something about the young man was familiar. *Wait . . . was that . . . ?* I could hardly believe it—it was my brother! I rolled down the window and shouted, "Jeremy! Jeremy!"

Let me reiterate, it was the middle of the night and pouring rain. New Brunswick is indeed a small city, but running into someone you know like this was highly unusual—having it be your brother, whom you see but a few times a year—seemed downright impossible. But then, this whole night felt impossible, so all bets were off.

Jeremy was just as perplexed as I was. He stared into my

window, puffing on his cigarette, trying to make sense of the strange girl in the 1986 Toyota Camry. I saw the moment of recognition land on his face like a revelation. "Jazz?" he finally said, as he ran toward my car and got in the passenger side—no doubt wondering why his nineteen-year-old sister was driving around New Brunswick at two A.M., weeping.

The rest of the night is a haze to me. We drove back to the Purple House, where Jeremy and I remained sitting in my car, and I told him everything that had happened. He smoked cigarette after cigarette. We were both drenched from the rain, both freezing. I put the heat on, and we just sat there in silence warming up, thawing our hands and our hearts. After about twenty minutes, Jeremy asked me—quite chivalrously and calmly, actually—if he could please get a bunch of his friends and go beat the hell out of Richard. I managed to laugh, suddenly—perhaps inappropriately—finding the whole thing very Sharks-and-Jets. I touched Jeremy's knee and thanked him, then said no, absolutely not.

"I could, Jazz," he told me, slowly shaking his head left to right, staring determinedly out the window.

"I know, Jer." I wasn't crying anymore, but a fresh devastation nonetheless settled in. I knew full well that things would always be different now, and that a piece of me would forever remain on Richard's porch, and in Richard's story. "I know you could. But . . . don't," I told my brother. "He's probably crazy. Who knows if he has a gun?"

And so Jeremy didn't beat him up. But the fact that he even asked—that he wanted to—was something that I would always remember as the moment when I knew that my brother absolutely loved me.

And that was all I was really looking for.

SIX

---

where the whole world
seemed to start

The next morning, I went to Planned Parenthood to get the morning-after pill. I sat in the waiting room and overheard one young woman talking to another. "This is, like, my ninth abortion," she said, then guffawed.

Where was I?

"Singer? Jasmin Singer?" The young woman with a tight ponytail working behind the desk called me over and asked me why I was there. I was standing in the middle of the waiting room, still very much in earshot of the other people there.

"Sorry?" I asked, wondering if this was really happening—if she honestly expected me to announce, in front of a roomful of strangers, that I had maybe, probably, definitely been date-raped the previous evening.

"Why. Are. You. Here?" The receptionist questioned again—punching each word impatiently, making her point even clearer with a punctuated snap of her gum and a widening of her eyes.

"I need to speak to a nurse," I said softly.

"Why?" she repeated, still at full volume.

"Excuse me?" *Was this really happening?*

"Why do you need to speak to a nurse?" she asked again.

That was when I whispered, "I think I was date-raped. I want the morning-after pill."

The woman behind the desk snapped her gum one final time, then just stared at me for a few awkward seconds. She kept her gaze on me, and I found it difficult to read her expression. "Antonia," she yelled behind her. "We've got a girl here who was date-raped."

My stomach jumped into my throat when I heard her say those words out loud. There was absolutely no question that everybody in the waiting room had heard this receptionist's announcement. I instantly regretted coming in and eyeballed the door to see if I could make a run for it.

A second later, though, before I thought to sprint, Antonia emerged, a look of concern on her face. "Come with me," she said softly, and I did.

I decided not to press charges, which Antonia was hardly sympathetic about. And I guess I understand why, given that her job is partly to embolden women to say no and to educate the community that no means no.

"If you don't press charges," Antonia scolded, a few minutes later in her office, "he could go out and do this again to other girls."

Ah, guilt tactics. I was all too familiar with those.

I noticed in my periphery that there was a vending machine out in the hallway. I honestly wondered if it would be rude to excuse myself for a moment and grab a bag of Doritos.

I have thought about my decision not to press charges time and time again over the past decade and a half since that night. I have questioned and then re-questioned my decision, but I have never found the precise moment of clarity that I've sought. I realize that what happened was indeed date rape, and I know the harsh statistics on the vast number of people who are victim to this crime. I do not blame myself for what happened, but I can't let myself off the hook for my poor judgment in allowing myself to be there in the first place, when I had been clear with myself all along that I did not want to have sex with him. Pressing charges would have resulted in a "he said, she said" that I was not mentally prepared for during that particular tumultuous moment in my life.

My future activism would come to encompass women's rights and awareness and prevention of sexual violence. I would often think back to the night with Richard and feel fueled to educate other young women to take every measure they could not to wind up in that position, and what to do if they found themselves there anyway—or what to do in the aftermath. I would also encourage women to speak up about their own rapes, so that others would realize that they were not alone and that what happened was not their fault. Though I didn't press charges, what happened with Richard informed the rest of my life, and—eventually, after a lot of healing—it helped to solidify my worldview of compassion and my commitment to speaking up for those who can't or, for whatever reason, won't.

On that morning, as I sat at the Planned Parenthood in New Brunswick, eyeballing the Doritos, I was told to go into the exam room. A few minutes later, a middle-aged woman with tiny square glasses and a familiar white coat came in.

"Hello, Jasmin," she said gently. "I'll be doing your exam this morning."

"My . . . exam?" I asked. This was news to me, and I didn't miss a beat. "Sorry, I don't want an exam."

The idea of yet another person, even a doctor, penetrating my vagina was too much to bear. I wasn't even sure I'd ever be naked again.

"You need an exam if I'm going to do a rape kit," the doctor explained emotionlessly.

"I don't want a rape kit," I said, my voice finally quavering. "Besides, I already took a shower at the Purple House."

"The what?" asked the doctor, arching an eyebrow.

Gynecologists and I did not have a good history. I had gone for my first exam the previous year, at eighteen. Pushing past the scarring memory of my pediatrician's invasive exam for long enough to make the appointment and force myself to walk in the door, I'd decided that since I was sexually active, I needed to be getting annual checkups. The fact that I dropped my favorite ring in the toilet within ten minutes of entering the gynecologist's office should have tipped me off to how nervous I was, and, as it turned out, I had every reason to be. Moments later, with my feet in the stirrups and my knees wide apart, a medical student walked in, and my gynecologist awkwardly introduced us.

"Hi," I said meekly.

So as *two* strangers looked into my vagina—which was serving as a teaching tool at that moment—and just when I didn't think it could possibly get worse, my gynecologist told me I could stand to lose some weight.

I didn't respond. I just stared at the ceiling with the rectangular panels and I wondered how far out of the way it would be to stop at Wendy's on the way home.

I recalled all this on that morning at Planned Parenthood, while the irked doctor—whose time I was apparently wasting—pursed her lips and crossed her arms.

No—I would not be examined. I was tired of spreading my legs.

And so she silently wrote my scrip for the morning-after pill, and I dutifully took my dose.

Years after my debacle, when I was performing in an educational theater company that brought attention to issues such as rape and sexual violence, I confided in my castmates about my experiences. They listened patiently and empathically, and—through offering their shared experiences and helping me to plant seeds of self-love that I never knew were possible—helped me continue my healing. Throughout my process of being trained as an actor-educator and slowly opening myself up again, I learned that, refreshingly, many Planned Parenthood facilities (and similar ones) are indeed wonderful places of learning, havens for empowering women, safe spaces for people dealing with sexual trauma. I found that although some of my experiences at that particular Planned Parenthood were unprofessional and painful, there is, in general, a lot more awareness now, and staff are much better trained in dealing with sexual violence.

Shortly after the date rape, I called Timmy—who had apparently been waiting for my call ever since I ditched him a year and a half prior. "Jazz . . ." he said to me on the phone, with an exhale and palpable relief. "Jazz . . ." he repeated, not finding any other words, but not really needing to.

We decided to meet in the parking lot of a diner on Route 18. Upon seeing me, Timmy just stared. I suspected then, and later had my suspicions confirmed, that he was taken aback by the amount of weight I had put on since he'd last seen me. He got into the passenger side of my car and gently took my hand. We sat in silence, and eventually I took a piece of his bright blond hair and tucked it behind his ear. He leaned in and kissed me, and we were together once again.

That summer, after finally convincing my mother that New York was safe enough for her quickly maturing and reliable daughter, I resumed college at Pace University in lower Manhattan, continuing for my BFA in acting. Mom recognized the difficult year I'd had and was thrilled to have me excited about something again. Finally, I was a New Yorker! When my stepfather, Wayne, drove me to the Hotel St. George in Brooklyn Heights for the first time, a massive hotel-turned-dorm where I'd live for the next two and a half years, I felt suddenly lighter. Tears lightly streamed down my face as I moved into my new apartment and overheard the unmistakable Brooklyn accents of passersby—I was, I knew then, finally home, maybe for the first time in my life.

The view from my room was a sweeping panorama of the New York City skyline, with the towers of the magnificent World Trade Center front and center, just on the other side of the Brooklyn Bridge. Brooklyn Heights was quaint enough—with the nearby shop-filled Montague Street—and the subway, which was just downstairs, took only four minutes to get to Manhattan's financial district, where my school was and where the whole world seemed to start.

My roommate, Jennifer, and I became fast friends. She was a recovering anorexic—a teeny tiny slip of a thing—and had replaced her severe eating disorder with an obsession that her teeth were falling out. She'd wake up at night and run to the bathroom to make sure they were still there, intact. In the evenings, she'd ask if I was planning on eating a bag of potato chips— the sound of me crunching away inexplicably comforted her. The loud crunch of the chewing gave her some kind of a high and so I gladly indulged her.

When I moved in, I brought with me several dozen microwavable containers of mac and cheese—each serving in its own little disposable plastic bowl (apparently I was unaware that you could get food in New York). When I think back to the crap I ate then— the nutritionally void, highly caloric, processed, addictive foods, the only thing that horrifies me more than the heart disease I was actively training for is the inordinate amount of wasteful packaging I was throwing away. Each time I ate one of these bowls of mac and cheese, I created an entire bag full of nonrecyclable plastic waste—which I'm sure is still floating around the ocean somewhere, clogging up the world just like its contents had clogged my arteries.

Habit is a funny thing, and we gravitate back toward our well-worn relationships—such as mine with food—for a reason. Though New York gave me the brand-new start I needed, and glimmers of happiness began to glow inside me like the flickers of light that dotted the skyline, I remained completely unconscious about food, and ate it with fervor. I was indeed recovering from the previous year, yet my old, poor eating habits didn't budge. What I ate, even though it was always unhealthy, provided me with the warmth and familiarity of an old friend, and my erratic and disordered eating habits offered a bridge between my old and new selves. Simply put, it was familiar, and so I kept at it.

Each morning, I would either walk across the Brooklyn Bridge or, if I was rushing, jump on the subway and ride one stop to lower Manhattan, heading directly to the Stage Door Deli—located just across the street from the World Trade Center—and get a cheese omelet on a toasted "everything" bagel with a side of steak fries. I would then walk the couple of blocks to school and consume my breakfast quickly and breathlessly.

I recall a friend of mine, Regan, wanting to eat together one morning. We had just sat down in the theater office, where I often hung out. Regan realized she needed a napkin, so she left the office to go to the front desk and grab a paper towel. I was keenly aware that I had a warm bag with my meal in it, waiting to be ravaged. When my friend returned not a minute later, I had already consumed my entire cheese omelet bagel.

I often tried to downplay the amount I ate, the speed with which I ate it, and the obsessive way food constantly circled around my thoughts and my days. I would frequently eat in privacy—as I had as a kid—feeling 100 percent comfortable (thrilled, in fact) consuming bagel after bagel, bag after bag of Doritos, in solitude. I was careful not to let my compulsion show in public. So when Regan came back into the theater office with her napkin and her uneaten breakfast, and saw that I was taking my final bite of my enormous meal, she stopped cold in her tracks—I had been caught. There was no backpedaling this particular moment, and so all I did was look at the floor, mouth full of eggs, and mumble, "Sorry—I was really hungry." I was also mortified. It was as though she had caught me masturbating.

Then again, perhaps I wasn't hiding as well as I thought—even aside from what I ate. As much as I wanted to avoid it, my carefully constructed veneer was starting to show cracks. And Regan wasn't the only one to notice.

Enter Clara—an out lesbian and passionate feminist who took an interest in me when our paths crossed at Pace. It was as though she saw me as a fragmented puzzle that needed a visionary, someone to help put together the pieces a little, or at least find the corners. And she was on to something—I did need a bit of putting together, not to mention someone as unapologetic and proud as Clara to put some things in perspective and shake things up. I found her fascinating—a five-foot-one bundle of electricity, with wisdom well beyond her nineteen years.

Clara headed up the LGBT group at school and organized a trip to see a major production of Eve Ensler's *The Vagina Monologues* at Madison Square Garden. With its multiple monologues based on multiple feminine experiences—including everything from puberty to orgasm to rape to genital mutilation—the play spoke to me deeply. At one point that evening, one of the presenters addressed the audience of thousands with this simple request: "If you've been raped, stand up. Stand up, women. Let's not remain silent any longer. If you've been raped, please stand up and be seen. Be seen!"

I thought of what rape meant. I had always assumed it meant being thrown against your will into a dark alley and attacked by a large, menacing man wearing a hood. Or something like what happened to Jodie Foster's character in *The Accused* (which was based on a true story)—being gang-raped at a bar. I did not think of rape as a foolish and lost nineteen-year-old winding up, of her own volition, in the bedroom of a thirty-five-year-old homophobic man. In truth, I did not know if I had the right to stand up.

Clara knew what had happened to me. I had previously con-fided in her why I'd left the University of the Arts and what the subsequent months had looked like. So when we were told to "stand up," Clara gently took and squeezed my hand. I looked at her—this brown-eyed, curly-haired petite beauty with a heart of gold—and I knew what I had to do.

The thing was, I didn't like being seen—*truly seen.* I know that's an ironic thing for an actor to say, since I craved being onstage as unrelentingly as I craved an extra-large pizza—and when I was onstage, I was most certainly at my best. I was, in fact, some-what of a natural there—and at Pace, I was given the hefty roles to prove it (Queen Elizabeth being my favorite).

But, in life I was guarded, because to be not guarded meant to show people the egg on my face—quite literally. I had seen the unmistakable look of horror when Regan walked in the room after I'd inhaled my breakfast, and I knew that was precisely the reaction people would have to me if they knew how fiercely I needed food, how bumpy and lumpy my naked body was, and how deeply I loathed myself. I hid behind my characters and I hid behind what I ate. I basked in the safety of manifesting other people's stories while my own personal truth lurked in the dark shadows that no one noticed.

All around me, women stood. The number of women who stood was staggering. How was it possible that this many people in one space had been the victims of sexual violence?

I thought of the night with Richard. I remembered the sound of the rain falling as I said "no," and as he held my arms back and hovered over me. I remembered, too, Richard's repeated proclamations that I could have been a model, that my body was beautiful and supple, that I was perfect. These two thoughts collided like thunder in my head—how could someone who purported to love my body so much violate it so completely?

My body was not his. For better or worse, it was mine, and I did not want to let him—or anyone else—take ownership of me.

Standing up that night was, in some ways, just a tiny gesture. But I had Clara's hand in mine, and that gave me the strength I needed to take this important step in recognizing not only that I did not belong to Richard, but that I did not belong to that memory. So I stood up, with thousands of women standing up around me—with them by my side and me by theirs.

Since I had taken a semester off when I left the University of the Arts, I graduated a semester late, which means I graduated in December 2001, which means I was a student during the attack on September 11. My school was just a few blocks from the World Trade Center, and the view from my window at the St. George across the river was a perfect one for watching the towers fall down. I screamed as bits of debris flew over the water toward Brooklyn and sirens filled the air. I was running a few minutes late that day, so Jennifer had gone ahead without me, taking the subway five minutes to the stop downtown—and was already inside the building at Pace when the first plane hit, so very close to home. Late that night, she returned to our room with tiny shavings of glass on her face and a haunting, new vacantness in her eyes.

Timmy had slept over the night before, waking up early to take the PATH train to his job as a waiter in Jersey City. The train that Timmy took had left from the basement of the towers, a thought that paralyzed me until he finally was able to reach me on the phone—reporting that he had passed through the World

Trade Center and arrived safely in New Jersey not even a half hour before the first plane had hit.

Because of its proximity, my school was turned into a triage unit, and we were allowed back into the neighborhood only if we wore masks. The whole city and the whole world seemed to shut down. I was traumatized, like all New Yorkers, and even today I cannot linger for too long on my memory of the buildings collapsing right in front of my eyes, or I touch the spot in myself where that trauma still resides, and keenly realize how painful it still is. Obviously I'm far, far from alone in that.

Chances are, you have an image in your mind's eye right now, thinking of that day. You remember the news broadcasts, the American flags popping up in random places, the unending and heartbreaking profiles of the fallen heroes.

But what's absolutely impossible to capture in a sound bite or a news story is the feeling of the aftermath of 9/11 in New York City. For one thing, the city smelled like death—quite literally like rotting, burned bodies—which is also impossible to convey on TV.

But what was truly remarkable were the little ways that complete strangers banded together, in sometimes silent but sometimes overt ways, in the days and weeks to follow. In and of themselves, these instances were infinitesimal—nothing extraordinary. But, the thing is, they were constant, like an ongoing ripple on a stream. New Yorkers like me clung to these moments as though our lives and our souls depended on it.

Shortly after 9/11, when politicians, celebrities, and neighbors all encouraged each other to go on as best we could with our lives, I remember clumsily taking the wrong subway to an audition and popping out on the complete other end of town, then sharing a cab with two strangers who had also wound up in the wrong place (that kind of thing never, ever happens in New York). That seems tiny—and it is—but it is also illustrative of how readily we each had each other's backs. I remember the new slowness of the city— the way we all trudged through the train stations and the streets with a unified sadness, but stopped more readily than before to hold the door for the person behind us, offering a simple, knowing smile: *We are in this together.*

It seemed that as a city we were allowing ourselves to be seen. We were standing up and being counted. We were refusing to let anybody take away the heart of us. We were remembering our innate kindness and unabashedly touching others with it. We were starting the slow but necessary process of healing. We were rebuilding.

That unobstructed, focused kindness motivated and moved me. I would shortly graduate from Pace with my degree in theater, and I would go on to work for NiteStar—an AIDS-awareness theater company that worked with inner-city kids to educate them, with theater as the medium, about safer sex, effective communication, sexuality awareness, and combatting domestic abuse. NiteStar was the theater company I had been auditioning for right after 9/11 when I had taken the wrong train—I had gotten the part. And not only was it my first real job, but the actors and directors became my extended family. We worked together and slept together. We partied together and fought together. And at the end of the day, we tried to change the world together.

Being seen was the name of the game—you couldn't put your-self out there as a mentor to kids without being completely present in yourself. And so I showed up. I was thrust into a community of largely African American and Hispanic coworkers—communities that are generally much more accepting, even celebrating, of a fuller figure than I had previously experienced. The people around me could honestly not have cared less that I was larger than they were. And so, in the safety of their arms, I started my life as a grown-up, with my eyes wide open and my heart ready to begin to heal. If New York could rebuild, I most certainly could.

There was only one thing getting in my way, and it was heavy.

SEVEN

---

for someone her size

I t wasn't as though I hadn't tried to lose weight before. I was a master at attempting to shed pounds. Perhaps it's a genetic trait, because my TM—always a size four—was adept at it, too.

Some people inherit their mother's dynamic ability to paint (I did not). Some people inherit their mother's petite waistline (not me). Some people inherit their mother's preoccupation with physical beauty, or her unending search for achieving the absolutely perfect body. (Ding ding!)

The ironic part is, of course, that my TM in fact *had* the "perfect" body. Not that she saw it that way. Standing at five foot six and with her weight always hovering at around 120 pounds, Mom was the classic definition of svelte and beautiful. As a kid, I would hobble down to the kitchen in the early mornings—my hair sloppy, my pajamas still wrinkled and creased and still clinging to my body with as much determination as the sleep in my eyes, neither of which would let go of me. And yet there was Mom—fully dressed in the season's most fashionable garb, her face covered in perfectly applied makeup (down to the precise lip liner). Even her chunky heels or strappy espadrilles would be in place. She was a sight to behold.

And yet she never truly recognized her own loveliness. My memories of her were not that she celebrated being a woman and being beautiful, but that she used her high standards as a means to focus solely on what she deemed to be the imperfections—and to her that was pretty much everything. Her thighs were lumpy, her stomach not flat enough, her knees sagging, her butt too prominent.

Not that this kind of insecurity is by any means rare. Other than maybe a few Buddhist nuns, almost everyone can probably relate to this. It's certainly not a secret that our culture of overabundance and overconsumption rotates around the ludicrous and self-serving notion that in order to be whole and worthy, we need to be ever more beautiful. Even people without any pounds to lose fall victim to this unattainable goal, always striving for *something*—eventually unsure of what it is they wanted in the first place.

Still, there are differences between the thin and beautiful (like Mom) and the rest of us. While stereotypically beautiful women may constantly and vocally battle with the last few pounds, or the tiny wrinkles around their eyes, or the one scraggly gray hair that defiantly popped through their perfect dye job, it doesn't seem possible that they're completely blind to the status their looks award to them. I would venture to guess that even my beauty-obsessed TM was very well aware, at least on some level, that she was always the most put together person in the room—and so her obsession was to maintain, rather than achieve, that ideal.

I wonder if women who look really good, but harp on the negative anyway, simply have a different frame of reference from the rest of us. Maybe they really do think they look bad—or maybe there's more going on there. This isn't to say that they're faking it, or that focusing on the self-perceived "negative" is simply an affectation—but maybe they think that doing so reduces how threatening they may appear to the vast majority of us who are remarkably and genuinely imperfect. (It doesn't.) And, of course, being the "most put together in the room" (or the thinnest, prettiest, smartest . . .) probably becomes wrapped up in their identity—if they don't accomplish that, then who are they?

So, whatever the inner demons that drove her, off Mom went to Weight Watchers, making the company richer and making me crazier with frustration. I often wondered how the other women there reacted when my mother—a slender, gorgeous woman with no apparent ability to see herself—walked in the door and said, "Hi! I'm here because I want to lose some weight."

Mom would regularly swing by the grocery store to pick up enough Weight Watchers brand microwavable meals and desserts to fill our entire enormous second freezer, which sat like a lone soldier in our messy garage. She fed those Weight Watchers meals to me, too—such as a baked potato (why not just *microwave an actual potato?*) with low-calorie melted cheese, or a single-serving lasagna that became rubbery and hard around the edges when it was nuked (yet always stayed somewhat frozen in the middle). We ate these meals straight from their little, white, thin cardboard packages. For dessert, I would opt for the microwavable chocolate cake—but then a half hour after dinner, I would sneak down to the "diet freezer" and grab a couple more, popping them into the microwave and hoping that Mom didn't hear the telltale *beep beep beep* when it was sufficiently thawed.

Mom was always extremely busy, so even despite her preoccupation with Weight Watchers and her obsession with both of us shedding pounds, it made sense that she didn't have time for elaborate, health-conscious meals. She worked as an elementary school art teacher and also taught in both the afterschool program and, frequently, the summer program (or a nearby day camp). These are tiring jobs that start in the very early morning hours, and my hat goes off to her and to all teachers for their fortitude. My stepfather, Wayne—also a busy, working person—was no help in the food preparation department, having no idea whatsoever how to navigate around the kitchen (except for the sink area—Mom ran a tight ship, and Wayne's job, which he did with diligence, was the dishes).

The microwave must have seemed like a godsend when it appeared on the food preparation horizon. But, assuming there even is a way to prepare frozen food in the microwave that makes it palatable, no one in my family ever managed to master it. I was recently sharing a breakfast with my brother in Brooklyn, and he and I were reminiscing on the foods we ate growing up. "They were never properly cooked," he recollected, specifically pointing to his memories of large bowls of reheated pasta with sauce, which inevitably wound up with that delicate balance of blackened and icy. Jeremy told me that when he first went off to college, during freshman orientation, the upperclassmen observed that the food in the cafeteria was decent, but "nothing like a home-cooked meal," and Jeremy remembered being confused, wondering how it could possibly be *worse*. The food at college wound up being the best he'd ever had.

But the microwave was not the only culprit in our own personal food desert. Our kitchen counter was where Mom kept her Weight Watchers reading material and journals, in which she scribbled down what she ate and when. In our house, eating became seen as an activity for how to lose weight, not an activity for how to find nourishment or—heaven forbid!—satisfaction. I would venture to guess that, busyness aside, had Mom not been obsessed with losing weight, our meals would have been a whole lot tastier and, ironically, more nutritious. Perhaps my outlook would have been healthier, too, because living as a chubby kid in the shadow of a stunning and skinny mother who refused to realize how attractive she was is the stuff future therapy sessions are made of.

Don't get me wrong—Mom never, ever put me down because of my looks. It was much more complicated than that. On the contrary, she always called me beautiful, and I have absolutely no doubt she thought of me that way, and continues to think it. She truly saw me through the rose-colored glasses that every mother is issued at birth, but which, from what I've heard, many take off along the way. She never took them off when it came to me. But given her complete preoccupation with losing weight, it was, to say the least, perplexing to me how she could truly feel I was indeed beautiful, given my size and her obsession with thinness.

And even if Mom did, in fact, think of me as beautiful, she never hesitated to tell me how fat she thought *she* was, and how much weight she absolutely needed to lose. And lest you think that this was her gentle way of sending me a message, forget it. Her preoccupation with her size was real. It was all about her, not me. The hubbub was all about her self-perceived "flawed" body. Interestingly, on the flip side, when she would lose a couple of pounds (or, for that matter, a couple of ounces), she would come home from her meeting and immediately report to me her success, beaming ear to ear the whole way, as I ate a tiny Weight Watchers cake for the fourth time that day.

If I'm making it sound like it was all Weight Watchers all the time, I'm making it sound way too rigid. There were many times when she bounced over to Jenny Craig, or even to Nutrisystem, just to lose those dastardly "final" two pounds that Weight Watchers could never rid her of. Once she was, yet again, at her "goal weight," she would hustle back to Weight Watchers for the "maintenance" plan, only to gain back the weight and start the cycle all over again. There were other deviations as well. At times she would venture into support groups for people who wanted to lose weight, and she was always quick to buy the latest weight loss shake on the market. The weight loss industry had a devotee in Mom. She was their dream consumer.

To me, weight loss was a way of life, albeit one I had not learned to negotiate. Up until I was a young teenager, I had simply observed it—I had never actively participated. But I always had the suspicion—or more accurately, the *hope*—that one day my turn would come. Simply by being Mom's daughter and by residing in our yellow house on Anna Lane, this constant cycle was something I became wrapped into. How could I not?

It started innocently enough. "Do you want to go out for pizza with me tonight?" Mom asked, a glimmer of rebellion in her brown eyes.

I was sitting cross-legged on my floor, playing Super Mario Bros. on my brand-new Nintendo. "Yes, obviously," I responded, looking up at Mom from the TV screen. I could never get past level three anyway.

"Great. Come with me to my Weight Watchers meeting and we'll pop over to Luigi's on the way home."

Ah, that was her ploy. And it was a brilliant one at that,

because there was little I wouldn't do for the opportunity to stuff my face with a thin-crust, crunchy, cheesy pie flecked with spicy oregano and robust garlic.

Let me be clear—the pizza was not in her plans just to woo me. There was also the fact that the time in between one's weigh-in and the beginning of the following day was known widely among Weight Watchers aficionados and other regular weight loss program attendees like my mother as "free time." Free time, which was most definitely not part of the official program, was, nevertheless, the only part of losing weight that actually appealed to me, and it would, in fact, follow me into adulthood. It was that magical period of blissful denial when you told yourself you were "allowed" to eat an unrestricted amount of whatever crap you wanted, and, in your deluded head, it did not result in weight gain. You didn't have to count calories or quantities, nor did you have to record your food choices in any kind of journal. Somehow, according to this mythology, any future weight gain had absolutely nothing to do with this period of free time, when even the richest chocolate cake was miraculously free of calories or accountability.

It was simply *your time* to do as you pleased—a shining and anticipated evening of reward to commemorate a week of feeling deprived and overly managed by the harsh confines of a diet. Not only did free time reward you with the sheer physical pleasure of the foods you had craved all week, but it had the double impact of giving your brain a rest, too. During free time, you didn't need to think about what you were and were not "allowed" to eat. Your life was not being dictated by anything other than instinct—or so it seemed.

There was also the joy of anticipating the upcoming free time. If your weigh-in was Tuesday evening, then on Sunday and Monday you would think, "On Tuesday night, I can eat whatever the hell I want," and you would start planning your escapade. It was a beautiful, liberating feeling. It almost made the rest worth it—*almost*...

Mom's Weight Watchers meetings were just an eight-minute drive away, held in a room inside a small community center. At that first meeting, I trailed behind Mom by a few feet, feeling awkward and on display.

"Good evening!" the receptionist (also the person who weighs you in) chirped to Mom, grinning ear to ear, looking like she might crack if she smiled any harder. (Weight Watchers employees are always all smiles and sunshine.)

Then she noticed me, the chubby kid hiding behind her thin mom, with thick hair, and—I'm sure she was well aware—more than ample padding (the very padding that Weight Watchers banked on). At the sight of me, the receptionist's already high-pitched, New Jersey–infused voice became even higher and more singsongy. "Well, hell-ohhhh!" she said, clearly unsure how to talk to a twelve-year-old, using the same cadence you'd give a sticky toddler.

"Hi," I responded, monotone—fingering the VHS-sized Game Boy inside my bag, wondering if I could play Tetris here without Mom getting annoyed.

Mom was busy removing her earrings, her boots, her blazer, her neck scarf—anything that could possibly weigh anything and wasn't inappropriate to remove. She had already visited the bathroom twice to try to rid herself of any extra pee before the big weigh-in.

I felt the receptionist staring at me. We were both just standing there, doing nothing, waiting for Mom to be sufficiently undressed to step onto the scale. So I looked up at her—a woman in her forties with frosted hair and large, red Sally Jessy–esque glasses that were sitting too low on her nose. A second passed as we took each other in—she kept her smile the entire time, though it was clear to me that she was wondering how such a thin, pretty person had such a chubby, odd child.

"And what's your name?" she sang.

My voice remained flat and one-tone—trying to compensate for hers. "Jasmin," I responded, uninterested—trying to remember that after this sideshow was over, I would get to eat several pieces of pizza at Luigi's.

"Oh, what a pretty name!" proclaimed the receptionist, whose name tag, I realized then, said, *Hi, My Name Is Donna!* (It even had the exclamation point.)

"And what's your favorite food, Jasmin?"

(Wasn't this a question you'd ask a three-year-old?)

I decided to go for honesty, and so I responded "Cheez-Its," smirking just a little on the left side, for I knew that my answer would make her uncomfortable, just as my preteen chubbiness did.

After I said it, I could almost hear Donna's inner dialogue. *Ah, makes sense . . .* was what I imagined she was thinking, as she took in my bulging belly and fleshy cheeks.

"Yum!" she proclaimed then, shaking her head left to right, her eyes extra wide and her mouth slightly open—because, apparently, what I said was *revelatory.* I wondered if Weight Watchers trained their employees in overacting.

Donna leaned in, got serious. "Speaking of cheese, have you ever tried our cheesy baked potato, Jasmin?" she asked me.

Mom had lost a half pound, so it was a good day. On days she gained—even a few ounces—there would be a darkness in the air that evening, a desperation and a floundering that was most palpable during the "free time," when what was supposed to be a joyous, celebratory feast became filled with self-flagellation in reaction to the weight gain. But on days like today when she lost even a smidgen of weight, everything felt lighter and happier.

And so we sat in Luigi's and shared a large pizza and garlic knots, each of us forgetting for a few blissful hours that our bodies were even a concern at all. In that moment, we were not fat or thin. We were not being bullied by others nor by ourselves. We were not writing down what we ate into our journal, nor scheming how to sneak our next illicit snack out of the refrigerator.

We were simply mother and daughter—sharing pizza, sharing a moment, sharing a life. It was free time—it didn't count. And yet, it counted more than anything else.

I myself first joined Weight Watchers the following year, when I was thirteen and had had enough—or, more accurately, when my TM had. I had spent a great deal of time crying and yelling about being fat, then trying on everything in my closet several times—sure that there must be a flattering sweater or skirt in there that would take off thirty or forty pounds if I squinted my eyes enough. I also had masochistically attempted to try on some of Mom's clothes. "We're not the same size," she'd say to me when I would come into her room, tearful, begging to please borrow something—wanting desperately to look as good as she did, knowing that her clothes were clearly the answer. She had enough clothing to open a small department store and, upon my request, would look and see if perhaps she had an open vest or a one-size-fits-most blazer (unlikely) so that I could continue to grasp on to the foolish notion that Mom and I could share clothes like we shared free time pizza.

Unable to ignore my frustration with my body—and probably aware of her own discomfort with my size (which was beginning to conflict with her undying conviction that I was, nevertheless, beautiful)—Mom asked if I might want to go with her next time to her meeting, but this time actually join—as in, as a member, not just a Tetris player. By then I was frequently joining her anyway, solely to bask in the free time afterward (lately we'd celebrate Mom's weigh-ins with a bucket of crispy fried dead bird parts from Chicken Holiday). And so signing up myself suddenly didn't seem like such a bad idea. I wanted to lose weight more than I wanted anything else in the entire world (other than how much I wanted to eat whatever happened to be in front of me at the moment, which somehow seemed to erase, momentarily, my longing to be thin).

And adding to the pressure to look like the other kids, to fit in, and to please my mother, always in the back of my head, there was Broadway. I needed to be on Broadway as soon as humanly possible, and I believed I certainly couldn't be if I was fat.

Thus began a twenty-plus-year on-again, off-again relationship with Weight Watchers—counting pretzels, then points; carefully scouring labels, menus, and moods. I lost some weight by following the program, though I never lost anything substantial—certainly not enough to bump me out of "chubster" territory. But when I joined that first time, I started to look at food not only as something to overconsume, but as something to deprive myself of—or at least to strive toward that. The idea of food as nourishment never even entered my mind.

A few years later, at sixteen, I was bigger than I'd ever been, and completely ashamed to walk into the doors at Weight Watchers again, wearing my failure for all to see. And so Mom took me to one of her other go-to places to shed pounds and swallow pride—Nutrisystem.

The petite blonde who worked at Nutrisystem did not acknowledge my presence any more than she absolutely had to. Instead, she addressed my TM, talking about me as if I were a nonentity—a heavy, nonfunctioning piece of machinery in the corner. "Your daughter is obese," she told my mother, in the same tone she'd have used to announce that I got a B on my math test.

"Excuse me," I said, interrupting this conversation happening around me and about me, "but that's ridiculous. I am not obese." (Plump, yes. But *obese?*)

The woman turned back to my mother to respond to my statement, once again only vaguely acknowledging my presence, as if I were just an idea of someone—not an actual girl.

She continued, "Given your daughter's age and height, her weight indeed puts her into the category of 'obese.' But there are solutions." With that, she looked at me and offered a smile, which was as far from genuine as the one I offered back.

The solution that she spoke of involved the herbal version of a weight loss drug called fen-phen (fenfluramine and phentermine), which was said to stop the formation of fats—as well as control hunger and reduce cravings. The original nonherbal version of fen-phen was an option at that time, too, but our new friend, Barbie, advised that I was "not yet at the point of needing that"; she said the herbal (which was a combination of ephedra and Saint-John's-wort) would be just fine for me (or for "someone her size").

My mother was uncomfortable about the whole thing and not so keen on putting her teenage daughter on a magic weight loss pill. But I, of course, was intrigued. *In for a penny . . .*

So we left our Nutrisystem outing with a bottle of herbal fen-phen, neither Mom nor I uttering a word the entire drive home. In the car, the bottle sat in a little plastic bag on the floor by my feet, a reminder of my "obesity," and cold, hard proof that I needed a "solution"—which of course meant that I had a *problem*. (Or that I was the problem.)

It wasn't as though I didn't realize that my size was an issue—it was pretty much all I thought about—but I existed in this haze and daze between knowing that I was not like the other kids and feeling like I was absolutely the same, stature and all. So pointing out the elephant in the room—referring to my fatness as a "problem" that needed to be addressed with medication—resulted in my feeling both completely perplexed and thoroughly ashamed. I knew, but I didn't know. I wanted to be different from how I was, but I wasn't sure I understood, or was ready for, the repercussions of that.

Food was my salvation. And so the idea of changing my eating and living habits to accommodate the physical change I craved—to be thin—didn't seem like a viable option. None of the "diet" programs I tried—not Weight Watchers, not Nutrisystem, nor Jenny Craig, nor the laxative teas I bought at the drugstore—addressed my "problem" from a systemic level. What these proposed "solutions" purported to offer was the ability to magically make me thinner if I would follow a prescribed meal plan for a limited time or—as in the case of the herbal fen-phen—if I would pop a pill.

Nothing I did addressed the reasons I overate in the first place.

For one thing, there was the imbalance in my life that caused me to start using food as my drug of choice. But much more importantly, nothing I did addressed the overarching issue, that the foods I consumed were highly addictive and unhealthy—the opposite of wholesome. These were foods that were literally designed to make me continue to come back for more, and so I did. Some of these were foods that were, in essence, outright lying to me, by purporting to be "high fiber" or "low fat"—and pretending that meant something—yet secretly giving me the precise mix of soft, salty, and sweet that would make a person like me want to keep grabbing for it. What other thing in life was so inexpensive (or in my case free, since I was still a child supported by her folks), satisfying, and accessible?

I took my herbal fen-phen a total of two times and lost a total of zero pounds. Taking the pills made me feel like I was a sick person, like I was in the mental ward and being given my settle-down-now medicine in a tiny paper cup. I opted against returning to Nutrisystem, and I shook my head in disgust the following year when the original fen-phen was yanked from the market due to the fatal heart complications it caused. Herbal fen-phen was soon removed from Nutrisystem as well, since it, too, carried a stigma, as well as conflicting reports on its safety and reliability. It seemed that to lose weight, taking a magic pill was not the answer. (Breaking news.)

My teen years were full of attempts at losing weight—which were frequently fleetingly successful, until I would gain my pounds back shortly thereafter. Throughout high school and then college, I was always up and down, up and down—though those ups and downs generally bounced somewhere between chubby and fat.

By the time college was over, I was my heaviest yet (though not yet nearly the heaviest I'd become). Even though I was an actor with NiteStar, the AIDS-awareness company, it only paid minimum wage. And so whenever I wasn't there, I was busy pounding the pavement trying to get (higher-paid) roles—and I like to believe I was talented and savvy. My monologues were well rehearsed and fresh, I was astute at cold reads, and I knew exactly how to navigate the business side of theater—I sent out a constant cycle of head shots and thank-you postcards, and kept an organized planner to map out my audition strategy for each week.

The feedback I got from casting directors, agents, and theater directors was always extremely positive. "Well, you're definitely good," they'd say, their pencil pressed up against their lips as they were lost in thought—knowing just as well as I that there was no role for me. The fat girl parts were few and far between—the best friend sidekick!—and you can bet your bagel every plump aspiring actress on the isle of Manhattan was gunning for them.

Getting a role in and of itself, weight issues aside, is hard enough—the odds are seriously stacked against you. I remember reading that for every one hundred auditions, you get two callbacks. Regardless of the specific statistic, the point remains the same: it takes a relentless and monomaniacal personality to truly do what it takes to get a job in theater. Being fat and trying to get a role takes an already teeny tiny window of opportunity and makes it that much more slight.

My body, it seemed, was getting in the way of my dreams.

Recently, a coworker asked me and a group of pals what our superpower was—in other words, what are we absolutely fantastic at doing, that we can pull out no matter what. One friend said her superpower is the ability to truly connect with people and have them open up to her. My own superpower is that I feel that if I want something enough, I can manifest it—I can make it happen, or at least make a version of it happen. Even when I was an insecure, bullied kid, I was extremely driven about the things I wanted—such as theater and writing.

That relentless drive stayed with me throughout my adulthood. If I have a goal, I will stop at nothing to make it real. It's a type of monomaniacal behavior to which I attribute the successes I've had in my life. I am a taskmaster—a relentless, *get-it-done* type of woman. If there is an issue, I will troubleshoot and fix it. If you have a problem, I will find you a solution. If I want something, I will figure out a way to make it appear—or, at least, I will try everything in my power, my *super*power. (The opposite side of that superpower—my "kryptonite," my coworker calls it—is complete tunnel vision and obsession with people and ideas. It can become all encompassing, and that's not always a positive thing.)

In my early twenties, becoming a working actress was my absolute top priority. My entire life up until that point had been about getting up onto the stage. From the time I was a little kid, that was what I studied for and prepared for. It meant absolutely everything to me—I would have put my life on the line for it. I had the talent, the business sense, the ambition, and the gumption to make it work. And yet the thing that got in my way—my body—was, I felt, completely outside of my control. When it seemingly mattered the most, my superpower failed me. I had no control over my body or what I put into it. It was a runaway train, carrying me along for the ride.

EIGHT

---

the hungry me

was broke. Though I spent my days working for the AIDS-awareness educational theater company, the pay was pathetic, and even with the addition of my regular babysitting jobs, I did not have nearly the money I needed to live in Manhattan. When I saw a job opening for a theater director at a sleepaway camp in New Hampshire, to direct a bunch of privileged, hormonal kids in *West Side Story*, I applied—and promptly got hired. The pay was not too shabby, and I was in great need of a change of scenery.

The camp was nestled on a large lake in the midst of lush greenery. Many of the staff members were from Europe or Australia, and they had all known each other for years—their summers were regularly spent working at this camp. I arrived two weeks into the season, when everyone was already well into the rhythm of the summer. I shared a rustic cabin with the other specialists—the art teacher, the music teacher, the gymnastics teacher, and a random assortment of a half dozen other twenty-somethings all keen on teaching our precious young ones during the day and secretly drinking to excess at night.

Timmy and I had broken up again earlier that year, after a failed wedding engagement and a brief attempt at living together. The previous years with him back in my life had been full of breakups and reconnections, and after the most recent period of remaining together—the longest one yet—we ultimately realized that it couldn't work. We were, it became apparent, glued together by a senseless devotion that ran deep, and contained much love, but was ultimately rooted in fear and familiarity. As long as we had the mutual dependence of our love affair, we could each continue to ignore the pieces of ourselves that needed figuring out. We had become each other's crutch, but no longer grew within our relationship—unless you counted the substantial growth of our respective waistlines as we filled the flaws in our affair with food.

With Timmy gone, by the time I arrived in New Hampshire, I had no anchor—and no idea of the monsoon that was about to hit.

On the night I arrived, I lay in my tiny, creaky cot staring at the cobwebs on the ceiling of the cabin. All around me were other cots, full of my snoozing comrades—who had been little more than lukewarm upon my arrival. All these years after being the "new kid" in third grade, I was the new kid yet again, and the circumstances were not dissimilar. My coworkers didn't know how to react to me—a chubby, intense New Yorker with weird clothes and a clear perfectionist streak. I didn't fit in, and even on my second night at the camp, it was obvious to me that nobody else wanted me to. It was more interesting to have a person to pick on, kind of like another extracurricular activity—I was something to talk about on rainy days when the lake was closed for canoeing. More than once, the walkie-talkie radio I carried around with me—which my coworkers used to gossip on when the kids weren't around—was the proof I needed that I was indeed the topic of too many mean-spirited conversations. I'm not sure if they were too dense to realize that I could *hear* the insults they muttered across campus on the walkie-talkie, or if they actually wanted me to know what they were saying.

And what they were saying was low. The inexplicable to me, but hilarious to them, ongoing joke was that I was a "transsexual"—and that I had a penis. Aside from the disrespect that this gibe illustrates for the very maligned and still frequently misunderstood community of people who are actually transgender, there was no impetus whatsoever for this rumor—other than to have something provocative to focus on, something to create a divide between them and me. Many of the staff became obsessed with this notion, and Channel 4 of the walkie-talkie soon became the central spot to discuss it. The idea that there's something wrong with being transgender infuriates and saddens me. This was just another level of upset that these rumors stirred up inside of me. It's similar to when kids use "gay" as an insult, to mean "messed up." When the reality of the summer that lay ahead truly sank in—when I realized that I would be ostracized in such a hauntingly familiar way, and that my inclination to defend the transgender community would somehow make it worse for me—devastation flattened me like a steamroller.

Shortly after I arrived at camp, when some of the others planned a trip to a nearby swimming hole on our day off, and I managed to tag along, my status on the bottom of their totem pole was crystalized for me. It was a brutally hot, sunny day, one of those days when the blinding brightness makes it difficult to see. We found a spot to settle on an enormous rock, and we stripped down to our bathing suits. Mine was black, obviously—a one-piece with a scooped-out back and a promise from the manufacturer to make me look ten pounds thinner (I often wondered why I couldn't just put five of them on at once and—voila!—look fifty pounds more svelte).

I looked down at my body—a bright white, fleshy target hung with the help of gravity and reminiscent of the geriatric crowd at my grandmother's swimming pool club. The bathing suit indeed ironed out the two stomachs I always felt I had, hiding the deep horizontal crease across the center and instead giving me just one round surface—resembling the big rock we all sat on as we disrobed.

There were six of us, total—four women (counting me) and two men. The other women—all bones and breasts and sun-kissed skin—were clad in tiny string bikinis. The guys, who were naturally focused on these three women, were eager to help them put suntan lotion all over their taut bodies, and the women returned the favor—laughing the whole time.

I walked over to them, which was no easy feat, given the steep slant of the rock, which burned the bottom of my bare feet. Nobody looked up. I twisted my long hair into a knot on the top of my head and adjusted my big, round sunglasses. "Hey, guys?" I asked, as they laid out their towels. "Can someone do my back with the suntan lotion?"

There was a palpable silence, and nobody looked at one another. Finally, one of the women responded—just loud enough for me and the others to hear. "Ew," she said.

I looked at her, and she looked at her friend—and then the

two of them burst out laughing again, because it seemed completely hilarious to them in that moment to be spending their afternoon with a "fat tranny." They would look, but they would not touch. They would laugh, but they would not feel.

Leo, by far the nicest of the group (which is not saying much), finally stepped up—still not making eye contact with the girls, nor with me—and did a quick smear of the lotion on my paper-colored back, then promptly walked away. "Thanks," I muttered as I returned to my towel, five feet away from the others.

The group decided to take a dunk in the swimming hole, and asked if I would watch their stuff, and then I could go in afterward and they'd watch mine. What choice did I have? So I held the fort down while they splished and splashed beneath me, grateful to the novel I was reading for providing me a bit of company.

Eventually the others emerged, and so I took my place in the cool and calming water, playing that game where you see how long you can hold your breath underwater. The swimming hole made me feel weightless and alive, and, for just a moment, I breathed in the sun and the day with all the oxygen in my lungs and hope in my heart.

As I made my way back to the rock, I noticed everyone was getting dressed again and packing up their stuff. Upon spotting me, they informed me that they were tired of being in the sun and thought they might go check out some nearby shopping.

"Okay, I'll get my stuff together," I said, sensing an odd chill in the air.

They glanced at each other and took a beat. "The thing is," said the skinniest woman—an Australian with messy, curly blond hair that I had the inexplicable desire to play with—"we are going to go without you. That way you can stay and read your book,

114

which it looks like you're really into anyway. And we'll pick you up in an hour or two."

The wave of nausea that cascaded through my body when I heard I was being abandoned is irrelevant now. The way they didn't even respond when I protested and said I'd like to go shopping, too, is neither here nor there. The fact that they started to walk toward the camp van, which we had borrowed for the day, leaving me standing on the rock and dripping wet, is—well—water under the bridge. In the grand scheme of things that went down that summer, I feel like the rest of the story doesn't matter much now. I don't think it matters anymore that I quickly grabbed my things and ran after them, promptly tripping and scraping my knee as I tried to catch up.

As the van pulled out of the parking spot, I hobbled as quickly as I could, my scraped knee stinging, and planted myself just behind the car—not even remotely worried about being hit. The van screeched and stopped, and Leo opened the door for me, the slightest hint of regret flickering in his eyes, as the others roared with laughter.

I got into the van, not saying a word. I was still wearing just my wet bathing suit, which one of the girls found even more hilarious. I continued to stare forward silently as the van sped down the street. I realized that I felt absolutely nothing (except the burn of my cut)—and I welcomed that numbness.

Out of my periphery, I knew that Leo was staring at me. "Hey," he said, beneath the laughter. I didn't answer. He kept looking at me. "Dude," he said a moment later and a hair louder, still mostly drowned out by the rest of the group's guffaws. "Sorry."

My feeling of nothingness shattered. Tears welled up in the corners of my eyes, but my sunglasses hid them, along with the rest of the feelings that I tried with all my might to push away.

When we arrived at the mall, I waited in the van. I awkwardly put my clothes on over my suit and did my best to clean my cut with my towel and a bottle of water. I distracted myself from my sadness by digging myself into my book—this fictional world where everything was okay, and where I didn't exist and never had. An hour or so later, they returned to the van more somber than before, and we all drove back to the camp in silence. The next day we went about our routines as if nothing had happened. As if I was not forever an afterthought—or at best a joke—in their minds.

For days afterward, when I showered, my sunburn hurt—especially the streaks of angry, red skin on my back that had clearly never been protected by lotion. That stinging was a reminder to me of how very much of an outcast I was, and I was embarrassed for foolishly thinking I might fit in. Looking down at my naked body in the shower—the ripples and hills that formed their own scenery, their own horizon—I knew very well why I had been left behind. Once again, I had been too much; there had been too much of me.

The one person who treated me with respect, aside from many of the campers who I cast in *West Side Story*, who actually seemed to love me for taking them seriously and were committed to making the play spectacular, was the kind and quiet woman who cleaned the cabins. Her name was Nancy, and every day she wore a different, brightly colored bandana tied in the back around her long salt-and-pepper hair. Nancy was in her midfifties, and she made up for her missing teeth with a warm and genuine smile. When she looked at me, her light blue eyes with the wrinkly corners seemed to see into my soul. By the second week at the camp—

which in sleepaway language is equivalent to years—I had formed a sweet bond with Nancy, which was refreshing for both of us, since nobody else there gave either of us a chance.

If I wasn't hanging out with Nancy—sitting behind the cabin with her as she secretly chain-smoked and I consciously tuned out the noise around me—I was traipsing across campus to my theater, where I was in the midst of staging the play, featuring a surprisingly moving rendition of Maria's death scene. Maria was being played, of course, by a skinny, thirteen-year-old Jewish girl from Long Island, but she knew exactly how to sell it, and I was proud of the show I was directing—even if the rest of my summer was falling apart.

Looking back, I am certain that one of the things that surely kept me removed from the other counselors, both physically and emotionally, was—once again—my size, pure and simple. But I know now it was more complicated than that. While there is absolute truth in the fact that they ostracized me, I was not without fault in my own remarkable ability to alienate myself. I was painfully insecure about my size and keenly aware of those times when I was the fattest person in the room—which was *always*, during that sordid summer I spent in New Hampshire. So I entered rooms with the certainty that I would be disliked when I got there. I didn't always allow myself the chance I deserved—nor did I allow others the opportunity to get to know me. They were blinded by my fat because it was all I let them see of me.

In the aftermath of the swimming hole incident, it occurred to me that I should have applied for a job at a weight loss camp instead—a "fat camp." It seemed to me that when it came to changing your behavior, there was actually quite a strong benefit in being pulled entirely out of your normal setting—in my case, the hustle and bustle of New York City—and thrust into a wholly different environment. Perhaps if I had been working at a fat camp, I would have been able to seize the opportunity of being away for two months and challenge myself to radically change.

Which was precisely when the radical notion occurred to me that I could change anyway, even if this camp was not specifically designed for weight loss. Why not make it my own kind of self-directed fat camp, and radically change all by myself?

I tend to be a black-or-white person. There is rarely any gray. For me, there is no such thing as doing something half-assed, and I didn't see why this new resolution should be an exception. If I was going to change, then it was going to be big. If I was going to lose weight, then I would stop at absolutely nothing. In New York, my acting career was floundering. I had nothing to lose except pounds.

Of course, the one exception to my relentless drive had always been my weight loss attempts in the past—they were never anything more than half measures. In pretty much every other aspect of my life, when I put my mind to something, I was all in. But when this revelation came upon me at this camp in New Hampshire, that I could lose weight in a vacuum—in a controlled environment where I would live and breathe for the rest of the summer and have nothing to distract me except rich teenagers—a firm resolve came over me, and I knew it was there to stay. No more half measures. My coworkers might have tried to leave me stranded, but I was not lost. *I'd show them who was in control.*

Whenever the subject of anorexia comes up, I instantly think back to this summer. I am not sure if just one sole summer of not eating any food (and I'm really not exaggerating—I stopped eating entirely) constitutes anorexia, since anorexia is a disease that frequently affects people for long periods of time and my bout was relatively temporary (even if my overall disordered eating and disordered eating mentality was a lifelong struggle). But that summer, after it became crystal clear how dispensable I was, I made the bold decision to test my body's limits and to see if I could finally nip this problem in the bud. "There are solutions," I remember the Nutrisystem woman telling me, years before. Perhaps all I needed was a kick-start. No more food, no more problems. I was cutting myself off.

I did not wean myself off food—I just stopped cold. I still showed up for mealtimes—because if I or any other staff member didn't, one of the camp administrators hunted us down. So my routine was to get a cup of coffee with cream (my sole caloric intake, aside from the occasional lettuce with canned pineapple) and sit with some of my cabinmates (none of whom had been present at the swimming hole), all the while singing "Officer Krupke" over and over in my head as they chatted with one another. I was disappearing further and further into myself, and my *self* was disappearing, too.

The hunger pangs were the worst all through the first week. They were sharp and intrusive, like a baseball being thrown full-force at me. In the middle of rehearsing with my campers, I would feel the sting in my side, which spread to my back and then traveled up to my head, dizzying me. I would drink up to ten cups of coffee a day, and so I existed in this mix between buzzed and fatigued, starving and drugged. By the second week of my secret hunger strike, I could barely walk from my cabin to the theater— and so I began to allow extra time to get there, knowing I'd need to stop on the way and sit on the ground in order to regain my strength and overcome my dizziness.

Hunger is a fascinating thing. It can obviously kill you (staggeringly, it kills twenty-one thousand people every day worldwide), but in the process, something about experiencing hunger so voraciously can remind you you're alive. Aside from the physical hunger pains that I got used to—and even welcomed, to some extent, as if they were a familiar friend—the mental and emotional manifestations of hunger came over me like a bittersweet revelation. It's shocking, actually, how quickly my hunger became a part of my identity, separating *me* from *them*, but also drawing a distinct line between the old me and the me I was now—*the hungry me, the thirsty me.* The me that needed sustenance, but decided to find it in my own resolve, rather than in cheese.

Somewhat miraculously, while my hunger did its job, I managed to do mine, and the play was coming along swimmingly. My campers respected the professionalism I brought to the show, and they found it contagious. So as I myself was wilting away—physically and emotionally—the buzz about *West Side Story* was taking over the camp. I encouraged a safe and supportive company with the actors and would not tolerate anything less. The campers inspired me—as soon as they walked through the theater doors, they transformed from dorky pubescent kids to artists, and they began to take everything about the show seriously. I ran a tight ship—lines were learned, characters developed, choreography mastered, scenery perfected, and a damn good show was imminent.

My two obsessions that summer became not eating, and making *West Side Story* soar. Zeroing in on those two goals gave me the focus I needed to drown out my coworkers, many of whom continued to make fun of me while I was in earshot, or over the walkie-talkie when they knew I was listening. For the first time in my life, I was able to stop caring what they said, because I had much more important things to concentrate on—some of which were literally life or death. That was another thing that hunger did for me—it gave me something to focus on that was mine and mine alone. As long as my hunger was there, I had something way more important to think about than the current gibe directed at me.

I was becoming very sick and had to start to make serious efforts to hide how my body was breaking down. Two things in particular made it increasingly challenging. One was my constant need to run to the bathroom, where I would sit for a half hour at a time, absolutely writhing in horrendous stomach pain, having unending diarrhea that seemed to come from nowhere. And the second issue, which frequently appeared at the same time, was blackouts. It wasn't that I was fainting per se, but rather, I started to see large black splotches appear, and I knew that if I didn't quickly find a private place to sit with my head between my knees, I would indeed pass out.

Ironically, I became extremely in tune with my body as it broke down, noticing every pang, jab, and gurgle. So when the blackouts would start, I would quickly tell the pianist to please go over "I Feel Pretty" with the cast, and I would hurry myself to the bench behind the theater, the one I was sure nobody knew about, where I would wait out the blackout. The dark blotches in my mind's eye became bigger, and the time frames when they appeared, longer. Though on some level these blackouts frightened me, I became remarkably Zen about them—allowing them the space to have their moment. Disturbingly, in retrospect I think I found the blackouts to be some-what gratifying—a telltale sign that I was winning, even though I'm not sure I knew what game I was playing.

Of course, my physique began to change drastically, too, and at one point, the camp nurse—whom I had never previously spo-ken to—pulled me over to the side to ask me what was going on. I was floored by the compassion and concern in her eyes. "I'm just on a bit of a diet," I said. And she left me to my devices.

Nancy noticed, too, and was somewhat in awe of my noticeably thinner self. We sat behind the cabin and she told me I looked good in shorts and wondered if maybe she should wear shorts, too. "You should," I told her. "They'd look nice on you. And besides, it's so hot out these days."

"You just look really good in shorts," she reiterated—more fascinated with my weight change than concerned by it.

She took another puff of her cigarette and we just sat there, staring at the woods and at the water just beyond them.

Soon my hunger disappeared, and my body seemed to find a new normal in its starvation mode. When I wasn't rehearsing or preparing for the play, I would find a quiet place to sleep—I was so extraordinarily tired all the time. I basked in my sleep, though, and was grateful for the opportunity to stop the world from spinning.

"You look like you need a break," the camp director told me one day, just before *West Side Story* went up.

"Nah, I'm good," I told him—keenly aware that I had large bags under my eyes and that, despite the unrelenting sun, my skin was still chalky and pale.

But he insisted that I take a day trip of my choosing and told me of a bus that went directly into Boston. I decided I would go, rationalizing that my clothes were swimming on my new body and I could stand to get one or two things that fit.

At Boston's Quincy Market, I popped into a store, eyeballing some jean shorts. When the woman working there asked me my size, I realized I had no idea. My unintentional uniform had become shorts or skirts with drawstrings, and large T-shirts. She looked me up and down, then suggested I try a six. I stared at her, waiting for her to add the *teen*—"six-*teen*." But she didn't. And when a six indeed fit me, and the woman assured me that their pants ran true to size, I was as excited as I was scared. Since I'd been a kid, I'd always been above a size twelve. It seemed impossible that I was suddenly a six.

I wrote to my mother, told her I'd lost some weight and could she please send me some of her clothes to borrow? The one pair of pants and one pair of shorts I'd bought in Boston didn't seem like enough. About a week later, a box of my TM's old clothes arrived in the mail, and as soon as I put them on, my new, thin body was as apparent to me as it was to my colleagues, whose comments about me seemed to fade as their curiosity bubbled— or perhaps I just didn't care to notice anymore.

One day, as I was gathering my things together in preparation for leaving camp the following week, I came across my box of tampons and realized I had not gotten my period since the first week of camp. That same day, as I was brushing my hair, a half-dollar-sized circle of hair—a huge chunk!—came right out, down to the scalp. It was just above my forehead, and to the right, and it was extremely obvious. I stood facing the mirror in my cabin, holding this very long, thick hank of hair that resembled a horse's tail, and I was terrified. I hid the hair in some tissues and pushed it down to the bottom of the garbage, afraid someone would find it. I fiddled with the rest of my hair and changed the part—figuring out how to wear it so that the new bald spot would not show.

It was finally the end of the summer. *West Side Story* was going up the following day. The camp director decided to take all the specialists out for pizza to celebrate camp being over, and I had no choice but to join. It had been a while since I had been around food, except for in the camp cafeteria. The toasty smell overtook the restaurant as we sat at the long table—me at the end. The director ordered a bunch of pies for everyone, but I didn't take any.

And as my colleagues around me ate their share and likely mine, laughing and joking about campers and summer memories, I felt a stomach pang again. "I'm going to get some air," I said, with nobody noticing—and I went outside, in the summer evening, and found a bench.

But I quickly realized that it wasn't the familiar pang of starvation I was feeling—it was dejection. For the first time since I'd arrived, I was able to see myself as an outsider would. Something about being in the pizza place, amid happy people and hearty food, made me feel completely alone. I had protected myself—or so I thought—by alienating myself from the others' gibes, and I had pushed my body to its physical limit.

I suddenly recalled the pizza I shared with my TM when I was a kid, and the warm memory made this moment sting worse. The people in my life who loved me—my grandmother and mother at the top of the list—would feel shattered if they knew what I was doing to myself. The realization that they would want me to eat the pizza broke my heart. I felt as though I was somehow letting them down. The love I knew they had for me from afar, as I sat weeping on a bench in front of a pizza place in some tiny town in New England, burst my facade and my bubble. I knew I was sick.

West Side Story was completely fabulous. The kids cried with excitement when the first curtain call brought down the house. As they bowed, they put their hands out toward me, begging me to join them on the stage, but I shook my head no and kept applauding them instead. It was their moment. I did not want to be seen.

Just after the final curtain call, as the kids were hugging their kvelling parents, I grabbed my duffel bag and left camp for good. I needed my life back.

NINE

sell a story and play a part

New York City was waiting for me. It was the tail end of summer, and the humidity stuck to my body like wet glue. When I walked in the door of my apartment in Washington Heights, my roommate's jaw dropped. "Holy fucking shit," she said. "What the hell happened to you?"

No longer surrounded by my controlled environment, I started eating again—but my period did not yet return. My hair, however, started to grow—first a soft fuzz, and then, eventually, the spot was hidden by a dark covering that, although very short, effectively hid the baldness much more efficiently than my weird, uneven part. And even though I had been so sick and knew that what I had done could have eventually killed me, I still could not help but bask in my newfound thinness. And the knowledge that I had the power in me to stop eating—to cease a completely necessary bodily function—reinforced for me that I could do absolutely anything I wanted, as long as I put my mind to it.

That, after all, was my superpower.

As I started to eat again, my weight, naturally, shot up. Anytime someone transitions from complete starvation to eating *anything*, that is a given. Add to that the fact that the food I was eating was anything but wholesome.

That fall, my obsession became how to make the perfect grilled cheese sandwich. I glopped on enough butter (to both sides of the bread) to oil a car, and then experimented with various types of cheese, finding ultimate satisfaction in good old American—my childhood go-to. In between sandwiches, I snacked on cheese and crackers and rarely if ever consumed a vegetable.

My body and brain were so relieved by eating that my mental and physical addiction took over everything once again—they were driving the bus, and any glimmer of hope for balance didn't stand a chance. I justified all this by reminding myself how traumatic my summer of starvation had been, and *how much I deserved this grilled cheese sandwich* with the perfect ratio of butter to cheese to happiness.

And so it's no surprise that very quickly I had to donate my new "thin clothes," and within just a few months I had put on fifty pounds. At the time, I knew that I was getting fat again, but I was in absolute denial as to how much. I simply could not keep up with my body, and just as I hid my dark moods with dark eyeliner, I hid my expanding body with an expanding eccentric wardrobe. Eventually, I went on the birth control pill in order to jump-start my period. I had outgrown (so to speak) my role with the AIDS-awareness theater company, and thrust myself back into a world of auditioning and scheming how to become the actress I had always wanted to be.

When callbacks remained stale and my career stagnant, I decided to enroll in a monologue class taught by a quickly up-and-coming casting director—a short and fiery thirty-something who spoke her mind, but who sometimes didn't realize just how powerful words can be. When Goldie walked in the door on that first day of class—her gait faster and her focus more intense than even most New Yorkers'—I was instantly smitten. Though she stood at only five foot one, her small shoulders were held perfectly upright, her chest wide, and her pointy chin was angled straight out and slightly up—as if she was constantly trying to smell something cooking in the next room—giving her both height and at least the illusion of confidence. Goldie looked like a stylish, prettier version of Velma from *Scoobie-Doo!*—who, admittedly, had always been my favorite. Her short brown hair curled under that determined chin, and she had the captivating closed-mouth grin of a woman who was always plotting. Though not your classic definition of beautiful, I found her quirky and completely adorable, and felt the familiar pang of my teacher-worship begin to surface.

The other five students and I fixated on her as she practically jetéd across the room, stopped beside a little wooden stool that inexplicably commanded respect, and then turned around to take each of us in. She hadn't put her bag down yet, nor had she said a word. The first thing out of her mouth was a question, aimed at the whole group. "Do you want to know why you're not getting cast? Why you have the time to take my class?"

We just sat there silently, looking at our teacher, unsure whether we should love her, fear her, hate her, or all of the above.

She didn't give us a chance to decide whether we wanted to answer her question. Instead, still holding her large shoulder bag, balanced impeccably on her small frame, she addressed each of us individually, telling us—based on her first impression of our appearance—precisely what stood in the way between ourselves and our respective Tony Awards. Red Beard Guy needed to shave. Purple-Haired Crew-Cut Girl needed a dye job, "at the very least," Goldie added. Mom Jeans Lady needed an updated look.

I suppose I knew, on some level, what was about to be hurled at me. But even though I had my suspicions, when Goldie stopped at me, not missing a beat, pointing her finger in my direction and saying, "You need to lose weight," a knot I had only then realized was forming in my stomach was tugged tighter, causing me to jut forward a bit in my chair, feeling both humiliated and defensive.

"I just did," I bravely replied, referring to my summer of not eating—leaving out the part where I'd gained most of it back.

"You need to lose more," she retorted, surprised that I spoke at all. (Fat girls don't speak!) She put down her bag with a clunk, then looked back at me. "A lot more."

And with that, my new acting class began.

Two hours and ten minutes later, after class was over and I no longer had to pretend that what had just happened didn't affect me—I stood tucked under a store awning on the corner of Forty-fourth and Sixth and wept. Once again, my size was betraying me. Proving that my worst fears were true, Goldie saw me as nothing more than a walking blob of fat and would never give me a chance to wow her with my ability to sell a story and play a part. My role, she had decided already, was that of a fat girl whose body was holding her back from getting cast.

And the sad thing is, I have no doubt—nor did I then—that Goldie was right. She was simply the first person in my career to tell me the unvarnished truth, even though I had known it all along.

The following week, I found myself in the elevator with Goldie, on the way up to class. She looked as though she was happy to see me, like she had something burning to tell me. "I'm glad you're here," she said, touching my arm and sending surprising, unwanted tingles up to my chest. "I wanted to tell you that I do Weight Watchers on Tuesdays before this class, and—forgive me if this is forward—but I wondered if you might be interested in joining me?" (Forgive her if this was forward?)

Did my acting teacher seriously just invite me to lose weight with her? This was definitely not the conversation I'd anticipated having that day, nor had I considered ever rejoining Weight Watchers. I associated it too closely with my TM, who was still—all these years later—in a cyclical, nonmonogamous relationship with Weight Watchers, going back every few months to lose the few pounds that drove her batty.

And yet, I was oddly moved by the invitation, and intrigued by the idea of spending "alone time" with Goldie, whose brain was fascinating to me, and—despite her insensitive streak—whose effervescence was not lost on me.

I acted unruffled. "Yeah, that would be great," I said, surprising myself with my (admittedly feigned) imperturbable attitude, and she told me she'd e-mail me the information about the meeting.

Walking into Weight Watchers was a strange experience. Even though it had been a lifetime since I last was a part of the program—added to the fact that this time I was an adult in New York City, not a brooding suburban teenager—the setup was remarkably similar to the community center basement where I had gone as a kid. Inside an unused room in an office building, I first walked in to a "pop-up store" of sorts—where I found all the Weight Watchers brand granola bars and other snack foods displayed, along with the attributed amount of "points" for each item. Just beyond the packaged foods was the receptionist, who still doubled as the person doing the weigh-ins. And hanging out near her was the group's leader—a bubbly aspiring opera singer named Cadence.

After I was weighed in and given my start-up materials, Goldie and I sat together in the last row and chatted, waiting for the meeting to begin. She had apparently successfully lost sixty pounds on Weight Watchers—a fact that surprised me not only because she was so thin, but because she moved and behaved as though she always had been. She appeared to lack both hesitance and self-doubt. I decided I wanted to be her.

As I got to know her over the next few weeks, I was surprised to realize that I didn't just idolize Goldie, but I actually really liked her, too. We started to spend time together—I would stop by her office in Midtown for lunch; we would pop into the produce market Stile's, simply because we heard the fresh figs there were perfection; and, on my twenty-fourth birthday, she took me out for an electric night of dancing and drinking (we didn't count points for the drinks that night). It seemed inexplicable to me that she was hanging out with me and seemingly enjoying it, and I basked in this new friendship—deciding that my ensuing weight loss would be an extension of that friendship, a way I could prove to her how serious I was about both my acting career and my devotion to her.

So I lost weight, yet again. I counted points and dutifully wrote down everything I ate in my tiny journal that was full of attempted inspiring quotes and sentiments such as the thought-provoking "Never give up!"

Once my class came to an end, Goldie was no longer able to

make our Tuesday night Weight Watchers meetings—so I started to attend solo. One day, on the way to my meeting, I had to run into the drugstore that was just next to the building that housed my Weight Watchers group. I grabbed the eye makeup remover I had stopped in for and, on the way to the checkout line, became distracted by a row containing shelves of large bags of Snickers, Three Musketeers, and wrapped caramels. I had barely eaten that day—on weigh-in days, I ate very little for fear of a last-minute gain or a full colon that would throw off the numbers on the scale. Since my points for the day were unused (and plus, post-meeting time is "free time," right?), I took a deep breath and bought several bags of candy. I pushed the candy down to the bottom of my bag and headed to my Weight Watchers meeting, where I was cheerfully told by the receptionist that I was down one and a half pounds. I grinned as I sat in the back of the meeting a few minutes later, knowing that my evening was going to be orgasmic—complete with the buttery grilled cheese sandwiches I'd make when I got home and the bags of sweet candy secretly hidden in both my bag and my consciousness.

At home later that evening, I treated myself to a binge and felt, once again, the tingling satisfaction that started in my throat and moved its way to my extremities—circling around my body and then finally landing in my stomach, where my fullness gave me comfort and security. It was my free time, and I indeed felt free.

I continued this ritual week after week—not consuming much of anything on the Tuesdays of my Weight Watchers meetings, and then binging on sweets that evening. The rest of the week, I remained married to my "rules"—the Weight Watchers guidebook that dictated how many points and what size portions to consume, how often, and with what diversity, was my bible.

Meanwhile, I continued to audition—getting small roles here and there, in plays that nobody talked about and that weren't particularly good. In the evenings, I babysat, and I had a roster of odd jobs that would keep me busy, but my income needs were far from being met. This floundering was juxtaposed by the success I was having at Weight Watchers, even despite my free time excesses, and so one day it occurred to me to apply for a part-time job there. I was, after all, a "success story" for them—I had lost weight and, though not at my goal weight, I had once again become a "normal-sized girl."

To my disbelief, Weight Watchers hired me! It had all come full circle. I went through a rigorous training period and soon began my gig as the receptionist, weighing in nervous, jittery women who, if the scale didn't display what they'd hoped for, seemed to feel they had lost everything that mattered (except the weight).

I could relate to having everything to lose. Despite my position with Weight Watchers, I was still not at my goal weight—and not on what they call "maintenance." My own group's leader, Cadence, who had been the biggest proponent of my working for Weight Watchers, told me under her breath that I was close enough to my goal to take the job. When I responded that I was still, in fact, losing weight, she said that upon glancing at me, I *appeared* to be at my goal weight, and since this opportunity was presenting itself now, I should record my weight on my application as slightly lower than it was. "You'll get there soon enough," she said with a wink—it was our secret.

My real weight at the time was in the 150s, which for my five-foot-four frame, was higher than it should have been by Weight Watchers standards. Plus, I was twenty-four, and thus still in the "under 25" category, which meant that I was supposed to weigh even less than I would have been "allowed" had I been just a few months older. In fact, according to the chart, even with my little white lie, I would only have fit into the "normal" range for someone my height if I were a senior citizen.

Even if I hadn't been, essentially, a fraud, being on the other side of the Weight Watchers table would have been an odd experience. I put on the biggest smile I could muster, welcomed the people who walked through the doors, and—after they removed all outerwear, shoes, jewelry, glasses, and anything else they wanted to remove—I gently asked them to get on the scale.

In this moment when they were weighing in, their lives were suddenly in my hands—or so it seemed. Most people held their stomachs in and didn't breathe, trying very hard to defy simple physics and magically will their weight away by holding it in. Maybe the scale wouldn't notice! Of course, I could completely relate to that mind-set, as well as to the mind-set that said that prior to being weighed in, you had to visit the bathroom and force out pee that wasn't yet ready to emerge—*even just one tiny extra drop*. I would overhear women telling each other how hungry they were because—like me—they didn't eat very much on their weigh-in days.

My double life as binger and role model obviously could not continue. Because Weight Watchers wanted its staff to be an example of the program's success, it required that all employees maintain a certain weight. So in order to keep my job, I was supposed to regularly get weighed in myself, and my weight was supposed to be recorded on a brightly colored card that said *Staff.* I was already slightly above the absolute highest end of that weight, since I hadn't been entirely honest on my application form—a fact that terrified me. Starving myself again, as I had done at camp, didn't seem feasible for me, mostly because I didn't feel as in control of my setting as I had been there—there were too many variables now. Besides, I didn't feel I had the mental energy to reenter starvation mode.

So I decided to deal with this weigh-in pickle by not dealing with it—in other words, I never showed up for my monthly staff weigh-ins. I knew that my deception would eventually catch up with me, but I was buying time in order to figure out what to do. Plus, even though I stopped weighing myself, I knew from the way my clothes were fitting that I was slowly inching up again. Perhaps, it dawned on me, my free time escapades were catching up with me. Other than the free time binges, I mostly followed the Weight Watchers program, though, admittedly, I was becoming lazy about counting points—oftentimes simply guessing at how many points this or that would be, and only recording it in my book every now and again. In other words, I had stopped following the program.

Eventually, as I always knew would be the case, my boss (who was also Cadence's boss) found out that I wasn't up-to-date on my weigh-ins and questioned me about why my weight card had not been filled out in so long. I lied and said that I kept forgetting, and that I'd do it that day. That day came and went, and what I imagined was my imminent demise hung like a rotten (two-point) apple over my head. I needed to deal with it, and I needed to deal with it quickly.

Something had to happen, and fast. Figuring I could put off my staff weigh-in for another week before being questioned again, I stooped to an all-time low, asking myself the dreaded question: *What would my TM do?* The answer? She would join Jenny Craig.

And so I did.

Confiding my somewhat embarrassing issue to my mother, who clearly had a sympathetic ear when it came to losing weight, without hesitation she offered to absorb the cost of Jenny Craig (surprise, surprise), and I eagerly accepted her offer (surprise,

surprise). As I had hoped, Jenny Craig took the guesswork out of it, sending my premade meals to my apartment in a series of boxes that soon took over all the cabinet space in my tiny Manhattan kitchen. I followed the regimented program for a week and was quickly down several pounds. A week after that, I was down more. My weight was still a few pounds higher than what I had written on my initial employee card, but it was respectable enough that I would not cause any red flags to go up. Nobody questioned me when I went in for my weigh-in, and my Jenny Craig success allowed me to keep my job with Weight Watchers.

Of course, by providing its members with prepackaged meals, the Jenny Craig program lacked a fundamental tenet of weight loss, and of health. I needed a quick fix—a way to put out the fire—and I got that with the Jenny Craig program. But I was still consuming highly processed foods. Besides, in the long run, joining a program where all my meals were sent to me was simply unrealistic, as it never addressed the root causes of weight gain—nor did it teach me how to eat in a way that I could sustain myself without gaining it all back. Fundamentally, here I was at twenty-four, and I didn't know how to feed myself.

In truth, I found all my weight loss efforts to be unrealistic and unsustainable—Weight Watchers and Jenny Craig alike, not to mention self-imposed starvation. Even looking at my TM's patterns with both Weight Watchers and Jenny Craig of *joining, losing, quitting, gaining; joining, losing, quitting, gaining*—how was that a testament to these programs actually working?

The reasons I ate remained exactly the same as they had been before, and nothing I had done in my life thus far had effectively approached these issues from a systemic level. The impetuses behind my maniacal, obsessive food intake were, by and large, twofold.

First of all, I was addicted (and, no, "addicted" is not too strong a word) to processed junk foods—which, ironically, included many of the decadent Weight Watchers snacks foisted on me at my meetings. The box bore a bright sticker that bragged *2 points!* but Weight Watchers left the lengthy and difficult-to-pronounce ingredient list out of its marketing scheme. The very ingredients that were regularly found in Weight Watchers foods—the milk chocolate, the sugar, the oil, not to mention the preservatives and endless lists of additives and dyes—differed from the ingredients in the Doritos, Cheez-Its, and Twix bars that I used to consume (and still consumed during "free time") only in that they were formulated to be lower in calories by limiting quantity. They were as far away from health-promoting, whole foods as one could get—with the exception, of course, of Jenny Craig's insta-meals. Of course, if you ate only a small amount of these foods, as you were supposed to, you could lose weight and maintain that weight loss. But, as I said before, I was addicted. "Small amount" is not a concept that addicts understand. Once foods like that crossed my lips, there was no such thing as enough. Ultimately, by their emphasis on allowing a small amount of these foods, but limiting the quantity, rather than focusing exclusively on the quality of the food, these weight loss programs smacked, for me, of deprivation. As I discovered years later when I lost one hundred pounds and kept it off, true health comes from finding abundance, both on your plate and in your life.

The second component I was missing in my quest to shed pounds was a bit more amorphous, but nonetheless became the main ingredient I needed in order to give rise to an honest and healthy life. The truth is, even though my whole life up until that point had been focused around becoming thin, I never once took a step back to look at the bigger picture—what food actually was, and what that meant for me. I was, I would soon learn, completely unconscious about my eating. Not only regarding the unbalanced, toxic, addictive relationship I had to what I consumed, but regarding the glaringly obvious fact that eating is the most personal political act there is. There were much bigger ramifications to it than just my pants size.

These two facts—my food addiction and my lack of consciousness around what I consumed—actually wound up going hand in hand. But until I was jostled out of lifelong patterns—patterns that were, it seemed, hereditary—I would remain stuck in this unhealthy loop-de-loop that governed my days and my consumption habits. Facing the reasons behind my food choices would, naturally, prove to be painful. But it was nothing next to what it would be like to bear witness to the ramifications of those food choices.

That, I was about to learn, was a whole other animal.

II

what i gained

TEN

---

someone else's flesh

Back when I was a young college student in Philadelphia, the definition of "eccentric" as I had known it thus far grew significantly in its scope. It was the late 1990s—perhaps the first era not to have a fashion trend all its own—and South Street, where I frequently hung my hat at night, was bustling with oddballs of all stripes. Some were stuck in the punk scene—with pink, stiff hair and spiky black boots that weighed more than they did. And some were still very much living it up in the grunge era, not noticing that it, too, was over—comfortably sporting large flannel plaid shirts with Chuck Taylors on their feet.

Broad Street, home to my school and my dwindling innocence, was fast paced and busy with a mix of tight-bunned ballerinas and cardboard-coffee-cup-carrying businesspeople clad in smart suits and simple sneakers (which they'd change out of once they got to the office). Everyone, it seemed, had an identity. Even those not overtly wishing to make a statement were making one with their perhaps contrived blasé attitudes.

Being a floundering kid-adult only perpetuated my fascination with how others chose to define themselves—or how the world defined them without their say in the matter. On Twelfth Street, a buff white guy walked hand in hand with a tall and dapper black man. On Pine, a pregnant woman pulled her long hair back into a knot, then ducked into an overpriced baby boutique with organic this and that. In Rittenhouse Square, a grandfather with his pants pulled high watched and beamed as his tiny, pigtailed granddaughter hopped in a circle on one foot. And I watched, too.

As I soaked in everybody's identities, I craved one all for myself—something unique that would separate me from the rest of the herd. Something that did not begin with *f* and end with *at*. I wanted to dig deeper. So I went from watching to experimenting.

My friend Hazel and I were barely eighteen when we found ourselves in a living room belonging to four fifty-something gay men, all sitting around smoking pipes stuffed with tobacco. We were there picking up our friend Rick on our way to a fellow classmate's party on South Street. Rick, also eighteen, had recently found himself rooming with these quirky men—one of whom was a family friend—in a beautiful big house on Locust Street.

Hazel and I awkwardly stood there in our gaudy sequined ensembles—neither of us had been offered a seat—and the four men proceeded to have a knowing conversation about us with their eyes, darting looks, and condescending half smiles at one another. They all sat with their legs crossed in their matching leather armchairs, puffing on their pipes and clouding up the room with their smoke and arrogance. Hazel and I had our very own inner conversation going on—we knew that if we made eye contact with any one of them (or with one another), we would have started cracking up, so we each did everything we could to avoid it, as we waited for Rick to join us.

Finally, one of them spoke—each of his words drawn out like he had time to kill. "What are you chiiiildren doing with your liiiives?" he asked.

"We're theater majors," I replied nervously and quickly, trying to compensate for his slowness by picking up my own vocal pace.

"What yeeeear are you in school, chiiiildren?" said the same man, which inexplicably caused one of his comrades to guffaw.

Hazel answered, barely audibly. "We're freshmen."

This time, it was a different man who spoke. "They're eighteen, Larry," he remarked. "Can you imagine? They're. Just. Eighteen."

Larry—the first guy—took another puff of his pipe. "Theater students," he said to his peers. "Probably bisexual. Probably don't know it yet."

And, with that, the men all chuckled, as Hazel and I turned the exact same shade of maroon as their living room furniture.

I was definitely not ready for "bisexual." In fact, I found the scene I had been assigned in Acting Studio, in which I had to kiss my classmate Mandy on the mouth, to be unbearably difficult (each time I went in for the kiss I would break into a nervous and loud laugh), and bisexual—let alone out-and-out *gay*—was not something I had previously considered. The very thought seemed absurd and embarrassing.

But clearly I needed an identity, and fast—and anything that started with the letters *LGBT* or *Q* was firmly off the table. Soon enough—following in the footsteps of another classmate, Emily (a lesbian, ironically)—I decided to find my identity in food choices rather than sexuality and made what I felt was the bold decision to ditch meat. Seeing as how I already wore all black and smoked clove cigarettes (though never inhaled, since I was doing it solely for show), I reckoned that slapping the label "vegetarian" on there was the natural next step in honing my image.

Given my lifelong obsession with food in general and cheeseburgers in particular, and my newer one with Philadelphia cheesesteaks, becoming a vegetarian was a pretty bold step for me. Throughout my entire childhood, my birthday parties had been catered by Burger King—each little attendee getting a cheeseburger all to herself, with two or three for me. I found no greater satisfaction than the one I derived from biting into a smoky brown patty and a melty, perfect square of orange cheese between two buttery white halves of a bun dotted with delicate sesame seeds. As I became a teenager, my go-to became the slightly more substantial cheeseburger you could find at any diner you'd pass on Route 18—the bun a bit harder and crunchier than the ones at Burger King, the patty blacker and thicker. A grown-up burger.

Within weeks of moving to Philadelphia to start college, I had already quickly become a regular at the cheesesteak food cart on my corner—trading in my fascination with cheeseburgers for their kitschier first cousin. The white buns, long ovals this time, filled with stringy brown meat intertwined with a gooey white cheese, made me feel comforted and sated. It got to the point where the guy at the cheesesteak cart I passed each morning—located on the corner of Broad and Walnut, just steps from my asbestos-laden theater class—would see me coming, give a little wave that I would return, and promptly start making my "regular."

Jumping from that kind of meat consumption to vegetarianism was a huge leap, and had I thought about it for more than the three seconds I devoted to this decision, I probably would have convinced myself not to do it. I'm sure I would have eventually landed on the side of plants anyway, but I'm grateful that I trusted my instincts when I did.

I went vegetarian for two main reasons.

First, there was Emily—my adorable, short-haired, baby butch friend, who had a painting on her wall of a naked woman (which always embarrassed me). Emily's vegetarianism seemed so sophisticated to me, her nonchalant attitude about it even more fascinating. Despite her decision to not eat meat, she still joined the rest of our group when we'd jaunt over to Johnny Rockets on South Street—and her hippie burger didn't look that different from ours. It was still blackened and crunchy, still encased in a thick white bun, still doused in ketchup and mustard, still served alongside salty fries. So, Johnny Rockets: *check*. I was in awe of Emily's ability to so seamlessly weave her vegetarianism into her life. It was simply a part of her, as fixed as her lesbianism or her light brown hair. It was woven into her identity. She *had* an identity. I was envious.

It was not as though I was after Emily's identity per se, but I was indeed after *an* identity. And the best part about Emily's was that it was a nonissue. Her vegetarianism (and her lesbianism, for that matter) was simply part of who she was, but not anything she felt the need to flaunt, or something she felt required validation. For me, even waking up in the morning required someone to reassure me that it was an appropriate thing to do, then someone else to congratulate me for doing so. Emily oozed confidence in a way that most middle-aged people haven't wrapped their heads around, let alone floundering nineteen-year-olds, and that captivated me. She was comfortable in her own skin, and I wondered if one day I might be, too. Specifically regarding her vegetarianism, it was not something she ever hit anybody over the head with, or even discussed very much. She felt it wasn't right to eat meat, so she didn't. End of story. I was impressed, and I was impressionable.

The second reason I became vegetarian was the fact that for the first time in my life, a food I loved actually managed to wear out its welcome . . .

Looking back on it, though I didn't realize it at the time, the day I ate my last cheesesteak was the first time I gave any thought to where food actually came from.

"Coming right up, Jazz," chirped the mustached man who made the cheesesteaks on my route to school. Though I saw this guy more consistently than I saw many other people in my life, and he'd actually cared enough to ask me my name, I'd never thought to ask him his in return. Our relationship was based solely on a sandwich.

"Thanks," I said, then proceeded to comment on the sunny weather—feeling that if I didn't say something, the only thing either of us would have focused on was the embarrassing regularity with which I consumed cheesesteaks. This was my second just this afternoon.

Walking away a few minutes later, I held in my hands my

three-dollar "home-cooked" meal. Why hadn't I known that food could taste like this? It wasn't even frozen in the middle!

Frequently, with my cheesesteak in hand, I would walk back to my apartment and consume it in privacy, or, at the very least, I would traipse over to Rittenhouse Square Park and eat it while sitting on a bench. But on days like today, when my appetite was ravenous and my energy frenetic, I would simply eat and walk, weaving in and out of foot traffic as effortlessly as I avoided the searing reality that each one of my sandwiches held inside the bun an individual—several individuals, more likely. Like most people, I pushed that thought out of my head entirely, choosing to ignore the painful truth behind the meat I ate.

But on this day, for some reason, reality intruded. I thought of Emily and her quiet boycott. I didn't even know the driving force behind her vegetarianism—whether it was based on health concerns, animal welfare, or environmentalism—but something about her decision to forgo flesh spoke to me in a way that, suddenly, I could not ignore.

With my sandwich in my hand and these thoughts occupying my brain space, I furiously walked across Broad Street, nearly tripping over my own feet more than once. I suddenly realized I was right in front of my school's main building, and the cascade of stone stairs leading up to the entrance called to my tired body, so I parked myself and my meal there. I had taken only a few bites out of my cheesesteak by then, and I was still holding it, tightly grasped in my hand like a piece of evidence that shocked the jury. (Was I on the witness stand? "Yes, Your Honor—I watched as this individual's flesh was chopped up and cooked by a person who then served it to me with a soda.")

An unfamiliar feeling washed over me like a wave, giving me a vague sensation of carsickness. I stared at my sandwich, but resisted the urge to go in for the kill—that is, to take another bite. Suddenly I realized what I was feeling, and the magnitude of it made me shudder. It was completely foreign to me, yet as soon as I realized what it was, there was no doubt: *It was the feeling of losing my appetite.*

"Holy shit," I said to the sandwich and to the ghost of Emily's influence. I eyeballed the pebbly brown and mucousy white innards of my sandwich, and it suddenly didn't seem like food to me.

More than anything else, the impetus for my vegetarianism was precisely that: the sudden, lingering realization that meat was, by definition, not my food, but someone else's flesh and organs. Not exactly a news story, I know, but it was a reality I had only glossed over before, accepting meat consumption as "normal" without even thinking to examine what that meant. I knew nothing about meat production, nor would I care to learn for many years, but the visceral reality that I was eating somebody else's flesh suddenly made me want to retch.

As I sat on the steps at the University of the Arts, I thought of my family cat, Rocky, who was the most remarkable creature I'd known. I allowed these images of my kitty, whom I missed fiercely, to assuage the angst of the moment. I smiled to myself as I remembered hanging out in the finished basement of our house on Anna Lane, then snapping my fingers two times, only to hear an exuberant and cooperative feline—my Rocky—sprint down two sets of stairs to join me in the basement, letting out a throaty coo as he ran the many stairs to be with me. I *loved* that cat.

Again, the reality that my sandwich had been an animal—many animals, in fact, though at the time I didn't think of that—crashed into my happy daydream of Rocky, and I was repulsed. It was a simple, and visceral, reaction.

It is estimated that a vegetarian saves ninety-seven lives a year. It's a good thing I'm vegan now, because I probably ate my entire estimated "allowance" of animals before I turned eighteen. In retrospect, the amount of meat I so mindlessly consumed as a child breaks my heart. Aside from the negative health consequences of meat consumption, I gave zero thought to the individual lives behind my burgers—the suffering, the lives cut short. It wasn't as though I didn't know that meat was, by definition, a dead animal. But, as with most people, that fact began and ended there. Nobody around me was giving it any thought, and I didn't feel compelled to, either. And even if I had actually contemplated what it meant to consume an animal, I would have thought that the animal was there for the purpose of being my food—end of story. I certainly would not have considered the needs or desires of that particular animal—an animal who had, just like me, been an individual with unique experiences. And just like me, too—though in much more severe and radical ways—that animal had been seriously misunderstood.

Being a suburban kid who didn't have any idea what a cornfield was like, much less a factory farm, maybe I assumed that what I ate originated at the Foodtown down the street, magically appearing on the shelves with the wave of a wand. At suppertime, it was placed in front of me in much the same way that the evening news regularly flickered on the nearby screen as my family and I chewed our dinner. Like the news, my food was just *there*, waiting for me to consume, to accept it as is. The fact that there might be another side to things didn't even occur to me. In the midst of a toxic relationship with what I ate, the truth behind food would have been too difficult to swallow.

None of this really sank in as I sat on those steps; it would be years

before I would give a hoot about the politics or social justice implica-
tions of animal agriculture. In fact, when I first became a vegetarian—
and for years afterward—I would only bring it up in conversation
by saying, "Yes, I'm a vegetarian—but not the mean kind!" Even
though the knowledge that the meat in my sandwich was indeed
animal flesh entered a new part of my consciousness, and abandoned
the section of my brain known as "denial" (where my sexuality firmly
remained), I was uninterested in converting others or in making "too
radical" a statement. I wanted an identity, not a bullhorn.

My friend Ronald approached. "Hey, Jazz," he said, not having any idea that at that moment, in my silence on the stairs, I
was going through what would become a massive life transition.

I looked up, snapped out of my inner dialogue. "Oh, hey,
Ronald," I said.

"I was just about to get one of those myself," he said, pointing
at my flesh sandwich. "Can't beat the guy on Walnut and Broad."

"I'm actually not hungry anymore," I said—which, I realized
as I said it, was the first time in my life I uttered those words. "I
took a few bites already, but do you want the rest of mine?"

Nothing like a broke college student to wash the blood off your
hands. "Hell yeah," he said, then he sat beside me and gobbled
up my indecision, allowing me the momentary space I needed to
fully digest the gestalt shift I seemed to be in the midst of. "I love
food you can eat with your hands," he continued, talking with a
mouthful of beef—and I meekly smiled, suddenly keenly aware
that the only cutlery in sight was the fork in the road.

Two weeks after going vegetarian, I ate a cheeseburger.

I was visiting my TM and my stepfather, Wayne, in New

Jersey, and we were having lunch at the Rainforest Cafe at Menlo Park Mall. It was Wayne who said that he didn't believe I could pull it off ("I'll believe it when I see it")—and, apparently, he was right. Though in retrospect it sounds like he was being unsupportive, the truth is, given the amount of animal flesh I had consumed up until that point, it was not even remotely surprising that Wayne doubted my commitment.

In that moment, I doubted it, too, so I ordered my good old standby—a thick, juicy, melty, substantial cheeseburger.

Habit is a force to be reckoned with.

But that glimmer of truth that I had felt on those steps in Philly shone through once again at the Rainforest Cafe. After I finished the cheeseburger, I felt immediate guttural regret at having rejected the newfound identity I had been carving out for myself. As someone who never, ever fit in—not even in my prestigious performing arts college program that was full of weirdos, pariahs, and queers (oh my!)—having a label that I could come home to and making a decision about who I wanted to be in the world was like a tiny piece of feeling at home within myself.

That was the last time I ever ate meat.

Of course, becoming a vegetarian did not quell my love of food, nor my ravenousness, nor my unrelenting appetite, nor my rapidly expanding waistline. It turned out that once I got over the initial emotional attachment to meat, ditching it was pretty much a no-brainer—and I simply flooded out my meat-centric dishes with cheese and eggs. Grilled cheese, cheese omelets, macaroni and cheese, and pizza became my new standard fare. (Not exactly health-promoting foods, and certainly not foods that are free of animal suffering—but it would still be a few years before I saw it that way.)

I changed the route I walked to school (I couldn't take the chance that my cheesesteak guy would see me—surely my newfound vegetarianism was negatively affecting his bottom line), and I became a regular, instead, at the pizza joint beneath my apartment.

When I told Emily I was joining her team, she winked at me. It took a moment for it to sink in what she thought I meant, and I became beet red. "No," I objected—a little too adamantly. "Not *that* team," I said, with an eye roll that I wonder now if Emily had been able to see through. "I went *vegetarian*," I continued. A moment later, I quietly added, "*That* team . . ."

"That's good," she responded with a salacious smile, squeezing my shoulder. She kept nodding and looking at me, giving me the feeling that she knew more about me than I knew. And she probably did.

ELEVEN

the most personal political issue

n case you haven't been paying attention thus far, my early
twenties were tumultuous years for me when it came to food and
body image. My vegetarianism—which I had embraced at
nineteen—simply came along for the ride as I left Philadelphia,
moved to New York City, stopped eating altogether, and then
reincorporated food and fatness into my life as though they had
both been lost friends (the toxic kind that you hang out with despite their smarminess and manipulative tactics—at the end of
the day, *they're always there for you*). But while vegetarianism was in
the background during my dramatic, toxic relationship with food,
it was, looking back, actually my constant throughout all of it, the
one part of me that was unwavering, even when the rest of me
seemed to be lost in space.

Another constant—at least for a while, after I had returned
from the New Hampshire debacle—was Smoochies. Smoochies
was a popular, low-calorie frozen yogurt chain that had locations

throughout Manhattan, most of which I was intimately familiar with. You could presumably eat a *vat* of it and keep it to under eighty calories—or, at least, that was how I interpreted the company's vague, at least to me, marketing materials. I ate something from Smoochies roughly three times a day—always making sure to get different toppings on my frozen masterpiece, just to shake things up a little. If you had cut my wrists, Smoochies soft serve would have bled out of me.

"I'll have a medium chocolate, with pieces of banana on top of it, and—why not?—hot fudge." I was at the Flatiron location at Twenty-third and Sixth, where I was a regular. Ice cream and its cousins (frozen yogurt, sherbet, sorbet) were the only things I ate relatively slowly (i.e., not at lightning speed), savoring each spoonful like it was rare art. I smiled to myself as I recalled my family trip to the ice cream place in Grandpa's van over twenty years prior—where I had also chosen to get chocolate with more chocolate on top. When it wasn't numbing or distracting me, food had the keen ability to transport me back in time, to happy memories of more food.

My watch beeped—I had a half hour to get to my audition in Midtown. I scraped my plastic spoon around the inside perimeter of my cardboard cup, just to make sure that I didn't leave any behind, and I made my way to my fourth "cattle call" of the week.

A cattle call is an open audition where all the out-of-work actors in New York show up en masse, then wait for hours in a crowded room for the casting team to call them in for an incredibly brief tryout. They are soul-sucking undertakings, and yet they are par for the course if you're insistent, as I was, on doing all you could to get a part.

When your name is finally called, you walk across a large dusty studio to stand before a table of tired casting directors and producers—"Hello, I'm Jasmin Singer, and I'll be performing a monologue from the play *Suburbia* by Eric Bogosian, where I'll be playing the part of Sooze . . ."—and then you throw everything you've got into what you hope is the performance of your life, as the timekeeper dutifully counts the remaining minute and a half until he can say, "Thank you—next!"

And that's that. Your afternoon is shot. You spent all that time doing your hair and your makeup, you waited for several hours for your moment, you finally got your two minutes—and before you know it, just as quickly as you are shuffled into the room, you're shuffled out. If you're like me, it's likely that the casting directors didn't even take you seriously, once they looked up from their notes and realized that you were what no audience (let alone director) wants: chubby. *Chubby, as in disqualified.*

But every now and then, while you're in the waiting room wondering how many more hours until they call number 235, you spot a familiar face in the pool of equally frustrated and hopeful actors, and you smile at her, knowing that at least you will have a friend to pass the time with as you waste your Saturday afternoon.

Sated from my Smoochies—at least for the time being—I headed up to Midtown to try out for an Off-Off Broadway play that paid a fifty-dollar weekly stipend. The studio was spilling over with actors, many of whom sat on the ground since there were no more chairs in the waiting room, and I had to avoid stepping on them as I made my way to the sign-in sheet.

That was when I spotted Marisa sitting on the stairs and reading the actors' trade paper, *Backstage*. I had met her through a coworker in my AIDS-awareness theater company, David, who was utterly enamored with her. It was obvious to me what had first caught his fancy. Marisa was your classic, all-American beauty—long blond hair, big brown eyes, full lips, and a figure that even models would envy. Yet there was something quirky about her expression, something endearingly comical about her mien, something surprisingly offbeat about her style. She was far from ordinary, and her staggering beauty seemed to be a nonissue to her. Unlike so many other beautiful women I knew, Marisa did not seem to notice—or perhaps *to care*—that she was the prettiest in the room.

"Marisa—hey!" I said, as I stepped over actors and made my way to her. She seemed genuinely happy to see me, and as grateful as I was to have someone to pass the time with as the audition gods ignored and abused our schedules.

"Jaaaazzzz!" she responded, like I was a long-lost relative. She closed her *Backstage* and focused fully on me. I squeezed in next to her on the stairs and got ready for what I was sure would be a long afternoon.

Admittedly, I was already somewhat fascinated with Marisa, even though I barely knew her. The first time we had met was at a picnic in Central Park. David had invited me to come along with them for this outing, which was a part of the weekly ritual following their Unitarian Universalist Sunday sermons.

I had arrived late and spotted David talking to this adorable blond woman who, even from ten steps away, was clearly extremely passionate about whatever it was they were discussing. She was wearing a light blue T-shirt with a pig on it that was captioned, *Friend, Not Food.* David had recently told me that his newest crush was a gorgeous vegan—and it was clear to me the moment I spotted her who this bombshell was. I got closer and realized the reason for her emotion: Marisa was lecturing David. It was in a playful way, but one that was nonetheless obviously and completely genuine.

"You'd better eat that entire sandwich, David, I swear to God . . ." she was saying.

"Okay, I am. I will," David replied, clearly as smitten as he was terrified.

"Those sweet tunas were killed and are now smeared all over your bread," she added.

And, with that, David noticed me standing there and introduced us—"Jazz, this is Marisa," he said, and I shook hands with the person who would change the trajectory of my life.

After the audition (I didn't get the part), I bid farewell to Marisa and treated myself to a thick, warm, soft New York hot pretzel—licking off each morsel of salt before even taking my first bite. It was the middle of the day and Times Square was full of eager tourists who walked too slowly for the fast-paced rhythm of the city. I thought of Marisa and how she was vegan. Before meeting her, veganism was nothing I had ever really given any thought to, and now that this new person was in my life, my gut reaction was simply to label it "radical" and push the whole idea aside. Despite the fact that I hadn't consumed meat in five years, veganism remained a foreign concept to me, as odd—I imagine—as rabid meat-eaters considered my own vegetarianism to be.

But when Marisa invited me to a screening she was organizing of a new documentary about animal agriculture, I decided to show up. Perhaps embarrassingly, up until that point, even though I was a vegetarian, I really had no idea about the issues involved with factory farming. I had never cared to take the time to learn, and I'm not sure that it even occurred to me to find out in the first place. I was comfortable with my decision to ditch meat and to leave it at that. I considered vegetarianism simply my own personal choice, an *identity* rather than something I would soon start to see as a moral imperative. I decided to show up to watch the film partly because I was being nice—I liked Marisa and wanted to be supportive of her event—and plus, I felt I already had a leg up by being a vegetarian. Then there was the fact that I was indeed intrigued by why Marisa had taken this "extreme" step of labeling herself vegan. I honestly didn't understand how it was possible to enjoy life as a vegan. It seemed so unnecessarily complicated.

At the screening, I sat on a hard metal chair with my ankles crossed. Just as I started to wonder where the nearest location of Smoochies was, the lights dimmed and dramatic music ensued. I decided to pick up the Smoochies conversation I was having with myself again later on.

It quickly became apparent that this film was not going to be the angst-ridden coming-of-age indie flick that I usually fancied—the only coming-of-age story here would be my own.

I watched as a former cattle rancher came clean about the horror he had repeatedly witnessed, the cruelty inflicted on animals as part of their standard, routine treatment—the horns, beaks, tails, and toes seared off, regularly, without anesthesia, in order to keep animal agriculture as "efficient" as possible. I stared in disbelief at the tiny spaces that animals were crammed into to live their entire, albeit incredibly short, lives.

Sinking farther down into my chair, I bit my lip hard as I learned that dairy cows need to be kept on a constant cycle of forcible insemination, then pregnancy and birth, in order to produce milk as continually as possible. It seemed so obvious to me in that moment that, like humans, and like every other mammal on earth, cows need to have just given birth in order to produce milk. I felt so stupid in that instant, as I half covered my face with my hand, wondering if others in the audience were also realizing this same obvious fact for the first time. I wondered, when was it that so-called efficiency had come to override basic humanity?

An image of my own mother came into my head—the bond we had when I was a little girl was still palpable for me. Despite our issues, we had always been close, and rounding that out, of course, was the very profound and meaningful relationship we each had with my grandmother, Mom's mother. The mother-child/grandmother-child relationship is a force to be reckoned with, and I saw no reason to believe that that wasn't true among other species. Who was I to decide, or simply ignore, what other species felt or didn't feel, thought or didn't think?

And so, when the screen in front of me showed footage of a dairy cow giving birth to her baby, and then having the baby immediately taken away from her, I felt my stomach begin to ache. This baby was off to face an uncertain future: Possibly this baby would become one of the millions of veal calves who are intentionally made anemic, often penned up constrictingly, and killed while still babies. Or maybe this baby would be allowed to live longer, in a miserable feedlot, to become beef. If the baby was a girl, maybe she would follow her mother into the nightmare of dairy production until, after about four years, her milk production waned and she would be killed to become fast-food burgers.

As I watched the film, right before my eyes I saw the mother cow bellow—she screamed—as her baby was dragged across the floor by his back legs. The mother's powerful instinct to care for her baby was completely squelched, and the baby's first experience was being painfully dragged away into a world of commodification and cruelty.

I had always thought that if you didn't milk a cow, she would die. I'm not sure where I concocted that silly notion, but I've since learned that it's pretty commonly believed to be true. As I grasped the jacket in my lap as if it were my own baby, I let go of the denial that had allowed me not to see the fact, now obvious to me, that the milk this dairy cow made was intended for her baby. And, unfortunately for cows, unlike humans, they can still produce milk while they're pregnant, so they can be forcibly inseminated immediately after birth and still be "productive." That means they are pretty much nonstop milk machines.

Milk had always been sold to us as kids as the most natural food on the planet. Ironically, however, humans are the only species to consume milk into adulthood and the only species to consume the milk of another species—a fact that, now that I was actually thinking about it, completely grossed me out (and it still does). As I sat there, it all seemed so surreal suddenly, and I briefly wondered if anyone would notice if I quietly exited this screening, this city, this state of heightened emotion, this world that no longer made sense to me. I desperately craved an out.

But just then, out of the corner of my eye, I spotted Marisa—dressed nicely in a skirt suit, a fierce determination in her perfect posture, her grounded stance. She must have felt my stare, because she looked over at me and our eyes met, illuminated by the flickering blue-green lights of the movie screen. We let a second go by with our eyes locked like that, and then she offered me a simple, single nod, which seemed to say, "I get it, I get you, and I've got you." I returned her gesture with a sad smile, and I let the new reality sink in for me that there was, in fact, no going back.

My thoughts lingered on the dairy cow. Though it was all disturbing, there was one thing in particular that I was thinking about obsessively—and that was that in order to produce milk, she is forcibly, repeatedly inseminated. *Forcibly inseminated . . .*

Intrusive images of Richard and that rainy night in New Brunswick came flooding back. I had told him no—my body was mine. But he was bigger, stronger, more powerful. And so he raped—*forcibly inseminated*—me. Over the years I'd thought about that evening, and I wondered if slapping the word "rape" on it was too strong. I had, after all, put myself in that position. But I did not give him permission to penetrate my body, and he did so anyway. In that moment with Richard, I had been there solely for his pleasure, and for him to act out his fantasies of power. What he did to me was an act of violence. I was a nonentity to him—a body, an underling, a vagina.

How was what he did to me different from what animals were forced to undergo? Images on the screen flashed before my eyes with the same mix of clarity and confusion as the images that flashed through my mind. Even though I was sitting, my legs trembled beneath me.

My reaction that night wasn't based on any intellectual understanding of exploitation and commodification of female reproductivity, both human and animal, although I would go on to read extensively about this connection in the years to come. It was entirely visceral. *This was just wrong.* At one point during the film screening, I surprised myself by standing up—jolting up, really—and then immediately upon realizing that I was standing, sitting back down. I honestly don't know why I stood up, except

perhaps because there was so much wild and furious energy cir-
culating inside of me that it was almost instinctual. The animals
on the screen in front of me made me question everything I
thought I knew about the way the world worked—the pigs in
gestation crates so small that they couldn't turn around; the multiple chickens crammed into tiny battery cages where their feet
would literally grow around the wires they stood on; the baby
male chicks who were of no "use" in the egg industry so were
suffocated in plastic bags, or ground up alive for pet food or fertil-
izer; the "beef cattle" hanging upside down, by one foot, after
they were supposedly stunned, though their bodies continued to
wriggle with life and their last bit of protest as they bled to death.
Each of these things—and more—was completely routine. It was
simply where animal products came from.

Any hopes that I clung to that there was a way to buy my way
out of this at some cute stand at the farmers' market boasting
happy animals and idyllic conditions were quickly squelched as
I learned that even in the most seemingly benign circumstances,
inherent cruelty is present. I learned that animals are never
treated "humanely," not by any normal person's definition of that
word, when they are commodities. The entire operation, the way
they are bred, born, and killed as babies, is simply not possible
without breaking up families. After all, virtually *all* farmed animals, not just veal calves, are killed after lives that are far shorter
than their natural life spans—their lives are measured in months
or even weeks. None of this is possible without forcible insemination (which is also pretty gruesome for the male animals whose
semen is extracted), nor is it possible without killing the animals
who are born with no "use" to their industry, such as male chicks
born into the egg industry. It is not possible to create animal

by-products such as dairy and eggs without also killing those animals who are considered "spent," like hens whose egg production is not at peak level, or dairy cows whose bodies are no longer able to produce milk fast enough. There is no reason to keep them alive once their peak is past—there is a constant supply of replacements, and their flesh can still be used for meat, though, of course, they don't fetch top dollar since their bodies are, by this point, tattered and torn.

My brain lingered once again—this time on the concept of families being torn apart. I thought of my own childhood, and my rotating family. I remembered how deeply I had loved my stepfather Brock, and how, one day, he was just gone—*poof.*

Still, despite my somewhat broken home, at the end of the day, I had a core group that I called my family. What would it mean not to have that? What would it mean to be born into a system where every one of your natural instincts and emotions are ignored and suppressed? These thoughts made me shudder.

It wasn't as though I didn't know that animals were killed for our lunches, our shoes, or so many other things that I didn't even think about. Dead animals were woven into every aspect of our lives. But the full picture and startling reality that was now staring back at me as I sat on my hands, trying to keep myself from jumping out of my skin, was life altering. Over and over again in my head loomed the question: *How could I not have known?*

Years prior, I had become a vegetarian because I was seeking an identity and because I had a visceral reaction to meat—it was gross, and that was that. I would no longer eat it. But I didn't think about the ramifications of the dairy and eggs that I consumed with clockwork consistency—making up the bulk of each meal and each snack I enjoyed. Until watching this film, it didn't

occur to me that even aside from the inherent cruelty of dairy—
the fact that the veal industry wouldn't exist without the dairy
industry and vice versa—and of eggs—the fact that the boy chicks
are killed at birth since they obviously can't go on to lay eggs
themselves—the animals whose by-products I was consuming
would eventually themselves be rendered "useless" and killed for
low-grade meat. I glanced back at Marisa, and, in that moment,
I kind of wished she'd never entered my life and turned it upside
down. *Goddamn pretty girls . . .*

But there was joy, too, in the film I was watching—and, refreshingly, there was unmistakable hope. There was the underlying
message that this nightmare didn't have to exist and that each of
us could actually do something about it by changing what we eat.
And, in footage that bypassed the brain and went straight to the
heart, there was evidence that, for a few of these animals, change
was occurring right then. They were getting out. Juxtaposed with
the horror show were images of rescued farmed animals frolicking
at a sanctuary, living out the rest of their lives peacefully and with
dignity. This was their refuge, and watching the film, it became
mine, too. Throughout the coming years, I myself would escape to
sanctuaries for a bit of respite and soul lifting, reinvigorating my
activism and reclaiming my own positivity.

Several years into my veganism, I met Rudy the Rooster at Coming Home Sanctuary in upstate New York—a small sanctuary for
rescued farmed animals, formerly abused and abandoned, who
were being given a second chance. It is operated by Laura George,
a fiery and quirky veterinarian with a big heart, who splits her

practice and her time between New York City and this incredibly rural area near the Finger Lakes.

When I first spotted Rudy among his flock of stunning hens, I honestly thought my eyes were playing tricks on me. "Why is that rooster wearing socks?" I asked Laura, who, I quickly learned, is the embodiment of imperturbable—thanks, I'm sure, to the mix of heartache and beauty she sees on a daily basis. Turned out it wasn't socks that Rudy was sporting—they were booties that acted as prosthetic feet. Beneath them, Rudy had stumps.

"Do you want to see how Rudy treats his ladies?" Laura asked. She grabbed a handful of blueberries from a small bag in her coat pocket, and Rudy, his jet-black and reddish-orange feathers glistening brightly, ran right over. Laura knelt down and placed a blueberry in his mouth, but rather than eating it himself, he gingerly fed it—beak to beak—to one of the hens. The hen ran away, pleased. Laura gave Rudy another blueberry, and he then passed it on to the second hen. This went on until all the hens were taken care of. "Sometimes it's hard to get him to eat," Laura confided. "He wants to make sure his girls are fed."

Rudy was rescued from a horrific cruelty case. He had been left abandoned, starving, bloody, and frostbitten. Laura took him in, carefully removed the caked-on fecal matter from his legs, and gently bathed him. That was when she discovered that beneath the debris, Rudy had only stumps—no feet. There were fragmented, fractured pieces of his toe bones embedded in his legs. He was broken. So she did her best to fix him, not knowing whether it would work.

Despite his injuries, Rudy took to his new home immediately— making sweet and sometimes piercingly loud rooster noises, nesting, protecting his flock, and charming anyone, human or not, who crossed his path. Me included.

When I think of the pain and terror that so many animals endure—animals just as vibrant and alive as Rudy—it can feel debilitating, as it had for me when I first learned what goes on for animals behind closed and bolted doors. Visiting Coming Home Sanctuary was a much-needed jolt of reality and inspiration. If sweet, chivalrous Rudy could rise above the system that almost destroyed him, anyone could.

I wanted to go vegan—there was really no other option for me, now that I knew what went on with dairy and eggs. You would think, given my lifelong addiction to cheese, that that would have felt like the stumbling block. But no, I was ready to let it all go—the cheese omelets, the Cheez-Its, even the cheese pizza. Surprisingly, it was my emotional attachment to my Smoochies that caused me to become momentarily paralyzed by my own indecision. It wasn't even so much the actual frozen yogurt product that I so enjoyed; it was the promise of consuming something that was purported to be so low in calories, while also tasting like such a decadent treat. I had come to rely on Smoochies for entire meals (now *there's* a well-balanced diet . . .), and it scared me to think about giving up that sense of security.

A few days after the screening, Marisa invited me to perform with her sketch comedy troupe. At the first rehearsal, knowing the emotional agony I was in about what I had been eating, she logically assumed I was going to do something about it and introduced me to her friends as a "new vegan," which stopped me dead in my tracks. For several years, I had been used to saying, "I'm vegetarian, but not the mean kind." And by "mean kind" (an interesting play on words, if you think about it), I clearly meant "not vegan," or, "not the kind of person who will make you feel bad about your lunch simply by existing." Was I becoming the mean kind after all? Now that Marisa had just thrown that label out there for all to see, what exactly did it mean about my life? Did being labeled a vegan mean that I had to grow out my armpit hair and wear patchouli? I was terrified at the permanence of it. I assumed that it was the kind of pedestal you fleetingly put yourself on, from which you would eventually fall. I was uninterested in failing at something so major, while everyone was watching, no less. Plus, *what about my Smoochies?*

(Speaking of Smoochies, there was a moment there at the beginning when I actually considered going vegan except for my Smoochies. And though that's laughable to me now, I have to hand it to myself for not letting my obsession with this frozen treat leave the door open to all dairy and eggs, during those first few days when I considered veganism.)

But Marisa mentored me, and within days I realized that 99 percent of my trepidation was unfounded and veganism was a lot easier than I thought it would be. One key factor for me was that I was immediately thrust into a community of like-minded folks who also cared passionately about their veganism and their advocacy.

For the first time in my life—and this was Herculean—I started to see food as something that was about more than just me. As soon as I learned what was happening with farmed animals—this bloody truth that animal agriculture will stop at nothing to hide—eating was no longer about my caloric intake. It was, I realized, the most personal political issue, allowing me the ability to vote with my dollars and my fork, to choose to either support or shun an industry that was reliant on my ignorance and my willingness to go along with the status quo, even though that status quo was destroying the planet and billions of individual lives in the process. I felt so stupid for having been so blind.

I also started to see animal rights as rooted in ideas that I wanted to have as the basis of my life—I saw it as an issue of fundamental decency and mercy. I have never described myself as an "animal person" and—except for my fond memories of Rocky and my firm adoration for my incredible dog—I would still not describe myself that way. I respect and admire animals but I don't have that *thing* that some people have that draws them to animals on an instant emotional level. My newfound veganism and animal rights activism was more about extending my bottom line of respect and dignity to the true underdogs: farmed animals. It wasn't so much about wanting to hug a pig as it was about wanting that pig to live her life free of oppression, and free from the machine that dictated when and where and in how much utter misery she would eat, sleep, shit, and die. Food, I learned, was so much more than just my own private battleground where I played out my daily struggle between desire and guilt. The idea that food was about so much more than *me* permanently altered the way I thought about it.

As this began to sink in, my obsession with Smoochies began to fade out. I was soon enmeshed in a world that was not only full of passion and purpose, but absolutely delectable. Turned out, vegan ice cream in all its incarnations was much more delicious than Smoochies. I should know: Throughout the next few years, I ate enough of it to write an encyclopedia about my findings.

I dove into veganism frantically and maniacally. I was equally obsessed with the reasons behind embracing it—which I saw as constituting a moral imperative—as I was with the food that defined it. The New York City subway suddenly became an elaborate web that unified the must-have vegan cupcake on the Lower East Side with the not-to-be-missed vegan "chicken" sandwich in Harlem, with the you've-got-to-try-it-to-believe-it vegan Butterfinger shake in Williamsburg, with the pinch-me-now vegan panini in Soho. I knew about all of it, intimately.

The "vegetarian" label that I had somewhat arbitrarily and thoughtlessly slapped on myself five years prior finally did what I'd initially intended—it became part of my true identity. It was veganism and animal rights that set me on the path to finding healing and purpose—opening up my love life (in my experience, vegans do have better sex), my social life (we're a barrel of laughs—sometimes we even talk about things besides castration without anesthesia), my taste buds (who knew that Indian food is so orgasmic?), and my life's mission (why be an unpaid actor when you can be an unpaid activist?).

It wasn't enough for me to just be vegan or to just be a part-time activist. I wanted this to be *my entire life*. It had never occurred to me that I would crave something as badly as I had craved being onstage, and yet my new life's mission—to dedicate myself to changing the world for animals—felt all encompassing, bigger than anything else. When I learned the truth about animals, I was outraged, I was furious, and I was on fire—and the last thing I was going to do was shut up about it anytime soon.

Nor was I going to stop eating vegan cupcakes anytime soon. Not only did this new stage of my life bring me into a world of passionate social justice activists, but it also brought me into a world of unending food. Needless to say, one thing that didn't happen when I went vegan was losing weight. In fact it was just the opposite.

TWELVE

opinions were for thin,
beautiful women

Becoming vegan and diving into a world that meant so much to me—animal advocacy—was the best decision I ever made. It gave me crystal-clear vision and purpose. How could I learn what was happening to animals behind closed doors and *not* do something about it? It was also a complete breath of fresh air to be working for something that wasn't all about me, unlike the work I had been doing (or trying to do) as an actor.

However, though my shift to embracing veganism and animal rights did radically alter my relationship with the world, as well as my relationship with food, it did not succeed in getting me to slow down or reevaluate my consumption habits. I was as mindlessly ravenous as I had ever been, and I justified my enormous appetite by telling myself that it was for the animals.

After seeing the film that compelled me to commit myself to helping animals, I decided to put all the drive that I had formerly channeled into auditioning into finding a job in animal rights. With the encouragement of Marisa and of her boss at the time, Maxine, within just a few weeks of becoming vegan, I went down to Norfolk, Virginia, to spend a week volunteering for People for the Ethical Treatment of Animals (PETA). If that experience doesn't thrust you full-force into the world of animal rights, nothing will. I see now that getting me a short-term gig with PETA was Maxine's and Marisa's insurance that I would be a keeper, and it worked.

Unlike the atmosphere at any animal rights job I've had since, the PETA offices had a corporate feel to them (that is, except for the many marvelous dogs and cats wandering around), complete with dozens of tiny cubicle workspaces, one of which was assigned to me for the week. Familiarizing myself with the antivivisection (animal testing) campaign I would be helping out with, I sat at my desk and watched video after video of chemicals burning away the cornea of a rabbit's eye, caged mice and dogs being force-fed large doses of everything from pharmaceuticals to household cleaners, puppies being bred to have degenerative eye diseases that culminated in blindness, and baby monkeys undergoing "maternal deprivation experiments," being pulled from their mothers in order to induce psychological trauma. As I sat in my cubicle watching a rabbit writhing as her newly shaven skin was burned with chemicals, I was incensed. I stood up to peek into others' cubicles and see if they, too, were fuming—or at least weeping. But what I saw instead was everyone typing away, working diligently—not unaffected (they had devoted their lives to work at PETA, after all), but simply *determined to make a change.*

Now that I had found my purpose, I saw no other choice but to be *all in.* And I was surprisingly successful. When I returned to New York after my short but life-changing week at PETA, I became obsessed with finding a job that was in any way centered around raising consciousness about animals. There weren't many, but there were a few, and so in the course of the next few years, I threw myself fully into no- or low-paying jobs, such as being an assistant at a small animal rights organization where I put together vegan starter kits for people curious about ditching meat; stocking vegan shoes in the basement of a vegan shoe store; and writing profile pieces, restaurant reviews, and eventually feature articles for a popular vegan lifestyle magazine. Eventually I even landed a position as the campaigns manager for a national farmed animal protection organization, Farm Sanctuary. There, I worked hard—extremely hard—all while I was fostering a side career as a freelance writer focusing on pro-animal, activist, and vegan-related stories.

I threw myself into this work with passion that left little time or energy for anything else. For me, controlling my food intake—even thinking about my food intake—was like a full-time job in and of itself, and I just didn't have the wherewithal. I also had a nifty rationalization that I hadn't had before: Limiting or scrutinizing my food felt like punishment, and unfair to do, when so much of my life was dedicated to helping others. So I figured eating to excess was my right.

It's become a bit of a cliché to associate veganism with thinness. The media certainly perpetuate this myth, constantly glorifying celebrities who jump on the vegan bandwagon for a few weeks in order to shed a few pounds and gain a few headlines. People also tend to think that vegans are all health freaks, existing on little more than leafy greens and steamed tofu. Though, more and more, the world is now catching on to the fact that vegan food can be as decadent, rich, plentiful, and delicious as animal-based meals, for the first few years of my veganism, the sugary, salty, and oftentimes fried food on my plate would have bashed anyone's preconception of vegan as a synonym for healthy.

The fact that vegan food can be so rich and decadent is a wonderful thing, since it means that people can leave the animals off their plates, and get them out of the factory farms, without sacrificing deliciousness. But—as with anything that is rich and decadent—vegan junk foods should probably not be consumed voraciously and monomaniacally—which was exactly how I was consuming them. In fact, my transition to veganism wound up being seamless—junk foods, once again, were central to my diet. There is literally a vegan version of every animal product out there, and so when I became vegan, I simply replaced the animal-based products I had been consuming with their vegan counterparts. While these foods are a whole lot healthier than the nonvegan versions (no cholesterol, for one thing), they hardly fit the myth that veganism, in and of itself, will make you healthy.

So, while the rest of the world may have assumed that going vegan would mean that my plate would be packed with nutrient-rich, health-promoting foods, like an abundance of vegetables, fruits, and other whole foods, sadly, that was not the case. Instead, I replaced my entire extra-cheese pizza (which was for me, and me alone) with the vegan version (I still did not share)—and even threw on a hefty supply of soy-based pepperoni for a kick. I ate salad-bowl-sized servings of macaroni smothered in cheese made out of cashews (which was unbelievably rich, creamy, and delicious) rather than cheese made out of cow's milk, which I was finally over, for good. Tofu scramble with soy cheese replaced my cow's-cheese omelets, and I'd be sure to have an everything bagel on the side with more than just a schmear of Tofutti cream cheese, plus a second side of fried potato wedges with lots of ketchup. Not only was my plate obviously devoid of vegetables and fruit, but in fact I never ate them at all.

But what really did me in was dessert. When I became a vegan, I was truly blown away (and still am) by the creamy, rich scrumptiousness of vegan baked goods. To say they taste the same as nonvegan baked goods would indeed be inaccurate. In my (vast, vast) experience, vegan desserts, almost across the board, far surpass nonvegan ones. (This fact has been corroborated by my opinionated brother, who is my reliable "meat-and-potatoes-loving" gauge and is unwaveringly truthful about what works—and, even more loudly, what doesn't work—vis-à-vis vegan food.) Of course, you can have crappy-tasting food of any kind—vegan or not—and not all bakers or chefs are created equal, but my expertise in vegan desserts (and, trust me, I should have an honorary PhD in this subject) proves that, most of the time, they far outweigh (so to speak) the dairy- and egg-laden counterparts. I was in a sugary, creamy vegan heaven.

Or was it hell? I felt as fully out of control and addicted to food as I ever had. I am by no means complaining about the fact that when I went vegan, I had the ability and privilege to fill my fridge and tummy with tall slices of the legendary-among-vegans Peanut Butter Bomb cake from the Bethlehem, Pennsylvania–based Vegan Treats, or with the plentiful variety of vegan donuts, pies, chocolate truffles, ice cream sundaes, or gooey brownies that seemed to blanket New York City with a sugary sweet glaze. These are glorious foods and should be savored—as should the fact that deliciousness and satiety can just as easily (and affordably, and accessibly) come from products that are entirely free of animal suffering.

The issue for me was that I was enslaved by food—both

physically and emotionally. So as I replaced my "regular" pizza with vegan pizza and my Smoochies with the cashew-based mint brownie sundae from New York City's premier raw restaurant at that time, Pure Food and Wine—while consuming virtually no vegetables—I also deluded myself that just by being vegan, not only was I taking care of the animals and saving them from abuse, but I was taking care of myself.

So, as I busied myself, round the clock, with my soul-satisfying work of changing the world for animals—and as I fed myself solely on processed junk food—the shape and size I came in was bigger than ever. And it kept getting bigger and bigger and bigger. Though my newfound work had given me the peace that comes with knowing that you have found your place in the world, my eating and my size gave me no peace at all. On the contrary, I thought about my body almost as obsessively as I thought about how the hell I was going to liberate all the animals in the world.

I was twenty-seven. I was at a friend's clothing swap—she called them "Bitch Swaps," which, radical feminist that I fancied myself to be, I found offensive—at her spacious Upper West Side high-rise. Many of her beautiful friends worked in show business or in fashion. They looked it, too. I was so aware of how fat I was, how my button-down shirt was pulling across my chest, causing a space in between the first and second buttons. You could see my bra through it—and I wasn't even wearing a nice one that day. I was mortified and, reverting to defenses I learned in high school, I was hoping that I had successfully created a distraction from my body by wearing extra eye makeup. I sat cross-legged on the floor, my arms in a knot across my chest, covering my wardrobe snafu.

The apartment smelled like Amy's vegan pizza, my favorite frozen variety, but I was too embarrassed to eat in front of all these skinny women who seemed to inhabit their bodies so effortlessly. I hated them—even though the better part of me knew that I shouldn't, that it was unfounded. I wasn't in high school anymore, and I didn't need to simply assume that these women were against me. I recognized the irony of feeling sure they were judging me and therefore judging them first. How were my own preconceptions of them any better than what I imagined about their preconceptions of me? Wasn't I just as much—perhaps even more—at fault?

I battled between feeling self-conscious and self-obsessed, knowing I was absolutely being paranoid. "It's not all about you," I'd recite to myself in my head. Besides, many of the women at this party were, in fact, sweet. One of them—a redhead with legs that ended at her earlobes—plunked down beside me. "Cool eye makeup!" she said genuinely, beaming.

I existed in a haze between self-confident and shattered. I spent my days working hard fighting for animal rights, and my work didn't go unnoticed. But each morning, as I caked on my eyeliner, as I put on just one more extra-glittery barrette, I felt myself sinking further into myself—into my fat rolls and my psyche, my bulbous stomach and my splintered self-esteem. Ironically, I learned how to digest the truth about animals, yet I felt traumatized by the truth about me. I was fat, and I spent every second that I wasn't fighting for animal rights convincing myself that I wasn't.

It was time to go around the room, show-and-tell style, displaying what we'd brought, seeing who wanted dibs on our stuff. I feigned excitement. I widened my eyes and pursed my lips in fake anticipation. Unless one of these women had recently lost half of her body weight and had some plus-size sweaters she was ready to re-home, I was confident that this was going to be an awkward afternoon for me, at best.

The first woman went. Size zero jeans. Hardly plus size, unless you're looking to outfit a Barbie doll. She got a taker, and lots of disappointed women were jealous because they weren't quick enough to raise their hands. Next, her size four jeans—"from my fat days," she said, explaining. I heard cutesy giggles. I giggled, too, because screaming at the top of my lungs to the point where my blood would boil and spill out through my pores all over my friend's expensive carpeting would have been inappropriate.

I discreetly eyed the balcony. I considered taking up smoking on the spot so that I could even momentarily escape this shindig, this mental ward, this cool kids club that I hated and wanted so desperately to join, all at the same time. All the while I smiled, trying to figure out whether I should pretend that it was cute to call your size four days your fat days, or whether smiling at that made fat-me look ridiculous. In reality, I wasn't even born a size four. Suddenly my TM's face appeared in my mind's eye, and I had the nauseating suspicion that she'd really dig this soiree. (Though she wouldn't have eaten the pizza, either.)

Big red hoop earrings were next. A few of the women, well-intentioned and kind, looked at me eagerly. One said, "Ooooh, give those to Jazz! They'd look so great with her black hair!" The others agreed enthusiastically—*too* enthusiastically. They were trying to ignore the elephant in the room—the elephant being me.

I exuberantly took the hoop earrings. "Oh, yay!" I proclaimed. Throughout the evening, I also took the guitar-shaped makeup bag, the silver and pink necklace that said *Fiercely Femme*, and the barely used turquoise eye shadow, which my friend accurately pointed out was just my speed. Unlike the clothes that got passed around from one thin person to the next, there was no question that the things I took home that night would fit me just fine. These items hit just the right note of ostentatious, too—a style I had carried on, in modified fashion, since high school, since I somehow felt that it effectively masked the parts of me I didn't want to show.

Not the earrings, though. I had never worn hoop earrings in my life. I just didn't like them. The ones I took that day, just so I could pretend I was excited about *something*, would be no exception. They would, however, remain in my jewelry box for years— a reminder of what those other women were, and what I was not.

The thing is, I loved the way I ate, and I had no desire to change that. It wasn't only absolutely delicious, it felt virtuous. And, whereas before I was eating the same few things (cheeseburgers when I was a meat eater, omelets and pizza when I was a vegetarian), becoming a vegan made me so much more aware of the possibilities of food and, as a result, expanded my culinary world in spades. Entire cuisines were opened up to me—Indian, Moroccan, Ethiopian, Japanese. And, aside from cuisines like those that were inherently vegan friendly, many of my comrades and acquaintances were totally hell-bent on "veganizing" traditional meat and dairy dishes, so I also regularly sampled more than my share of new plant-based cheeses, milks, specialty items like Faux Gras (replacing foie gras), and any of the barrage of vegan meats that were constantly hitting the shelves. To me, as a new vegan, food was no longer just my escape or distraction—it was representative of a worldview shared by like-minded folks all over the world. It brought me into a community that fought, against all odds, for animal rights, and then, as a collective reward, ate abundantly and purposefully. I loved that.

In fact, when I became vegan, I became a passionate foodie, and plant-based eating—in addition to becoming a moral imperative for me—also became a fantastic hobby. This happens to a lot of people who go vegan—it's an entire subculture of must-have yumminess. Tasting the most recent vegan products, and visiting the newest vegan restaurants or vegan-friendly ones, is just part of the whole scene. There are multiple websites and mobile apps (like HappyCow.net) that make searching for vegan food pretty much a no-brainer.

Not only did I live in Manhattan, which is a vegan mecca full of over 150 vegetarian restaurants, but I started to plan all my travel around vegan restaurants. When I was lucky enough to attend an animal rights conference in South Africa, I knew that the first place I'd hit up would be the all-vegan Greenside Café in Johannesburg. When I traveled to Vancouver, it was clear that the Naam, in Kitsilano, would be my mainstay, but in addition, every corner hot dog stand there offered a vegan hot dog (which, I'm sad to say, is far from the case in New York)—and so clearly that became my daily snack, multiple times a day.

During my travels, where I gave talks and workshops on veganism, activism, and writing for social justice, I experienced cities like Chicago, San Francisco, Toronto, Los Angeles, Philadelphia, and Boston as if they were jungles of vegan food—I needed to try it all. Sometimes I was in these cities for only one solid day, and yet I simply had to traipse across town just to try the cookie dough peanut butter shake at the Chicago Diner, or the vegan cheesesteak at Gianni's (now Blackbird Pizzeria) in Philadelphia—which, I might add, was a surreal experience. Just knowing that everything I loved to eat was available to me without animal products, and that there was a passionate group of change makers and foodies at the bottom of this food revolution, buoyed me.

In some ways, even though my initial veganism resulted in my gaining weight—and continued to perpetuate my imbalanced relationship with food—it also started me down the road that would eventually help me put that relationship in balance. What it gave me, immediately and permanently, was perspective. Prior to my veganism, I had been almost solely self-focused—when you're an aspiring actor, it's difficult to be anything *but*. Adding activism to the mix changes things. The animals for whom I was speaking were simply invisible to virtually everybody else, and so they relied on people like me and my comrades to amplify their voices. Focusing on that, instead of whether I was the fattest actor in the room at the audition, allowed many other things in my life to shift around, too, and ultimately to fall into place.

But though I was, in some ways, beginning to find my true self, it would be years before I would find balance with my eating. The fact that so many of the foods I chose to eat (actually, *all of them*) were highly processed, oily, and sugary meant that I felt lethargic and sluggish, much like in my meat and cheese days. Like a drug addict needing his next fix, the way I dealt with my fatigue was to eat more.

By the time I officially traded in cattle calls for saving cows, it seemed I had discovered this part of myself—my activist force—that grounded me at my foundation and provided my life with profound meaning and a productive outlet for my relentless drive. I stood firmer with my feet planted beneath me. For the first time,

I felt I knew who I was and exactly what I wanted to accomplish. And yet, despite that, even as I grew more and more self-aware when it came to eating, I continued to lack the fundamental self-care that I needed in order to thrive. I adored the food I ate, and nothing made me happier than eating it. But it wore me down, and my weight and size were as concerning to me as ever, as much on my mind as when I was in high school, making the dreaded walk to the front of the classroom for the bathroom key.

Looking in the mirror in the morning was always a painful moment, as was picking out my outfit for the day. Just like when I was a kid, each day I would try on multiple outfits, constantly convinced that the issue was with my clothes, and not with me. I would finally decide on something multilayered and eccentric, such as a sequined turquoise floor-length skirt—anything to distract the onlookers, anything to distract me.

My roommate, Rachel—a kindhearted performer whom I had met on craigslist and remain friends with to this day—would look at my wardrobe, wide-eyed, while eating her breakfast, and say, "Jazz, I have no idea how you put together such creative outfits. You look amazing."

I would respond, "Ah, it's nothing . . . just what I gravitate toward. But thanks!" and then, with a wink, stick my fork into a chunk of the potato on her plate.

Indeed, I had become a walking contradiction. On one hand, I was self-assured and confident—making my style seem as effortlessly put together as my attitude. But the shattered "new kid" inside me had never disappeared, and as my weight continued to shoot up, the still-broken parts of me began to crumble. I felt embarrassed for caring so much what I looked like—especially now that my life's priorities seemed so clear to me.

But despite all that, the plethora of food options captivated and controlled me. I craved it, both physically and emotionally, and—just as it had been before—food was always there for me to turn to. So I turned to it, again and again. And then one day, when I realized I could not climb the subway stairs without stopping halfway to rest, or partake in a relatively short fund-raiser walkathon, and when the only way I could get through the day was with regular doses of coffee and simple carbs, it occurred to me that I was eating myself sick.

"I have the worst headache in the world. Oh, my God . . ."

It was six A.M. and I was standing at Columbus Circle, just at the southwest entrance to Central Park. It was the day of Farm Sanctuary's New York City Walk for Farm Animals, and I was the organizer. In just a few hours, literally thousands of people would be arriving, registering, and walking through the park with signs celebrating veganism and raising awareness about the horrors that farmed animals endure. There were speakers, bands, organizations manning tables, information stands, goodie bags, food booths, and about seventy-five volunteers—all reporting to me. I was already on my third coffee of the day and would not be slowing down anytime soon. As I stood at the helm of this event, which ultimately would raise over eighty thousand dollars for the rescue efforts of Farm Sanctuary, I was a mix of jubilant and overwhelmed. Discovering my activism had been a remarkable experience for many reasons, one of which being that it brought out my inner community organizer, and—bossy bitch that I am—it turned out I was a natural.

On days like this one, it never would have occurred to me why my back ached, my head ached, and my feet ached. Politely excusing myself from the pre-event mayhem to grab a vegan muffin from the nearby Whole Foods, plus a second bagel and a fourth cup of coffee, simply seemed to me like fueling up to get through the morning. I didn't make the connection between my lack of real nutrition and my remarkable dearth of energy.

"Are you going to walk through the park, too?" The person asking me the question was clad in a cow costume. The kitsch of this event did not escape me—I found it charming and amusing, but also saw that the lighthearted approach to raising awareness was often effective. The point of this event was to celebrate, not mourn; to provide opportunities, not criticism.

"Nah, I have to hang back and get the food set up for when y'all come back," I told the cow, who nodded and walked away to join the giant chicken. I had been being honest with the cow, yet I left out the part about how I couldn't have walked the three-mile route through the park even if I had wanted to. Though I was in my twenties, my body felt like it belonged to someone's grandma.

As soon as the attendees were off walking on their route, I visited the nearby hot pretzel stand for a snack—then I popped a couple of Advil that I kept in my pocket to help my overall body pain and fatigue, which I simply accepted as part of my life.

Everything I did was physically trying. Even regular everyday activities like walking home from the nearby grocery store—which included a tiny incline in the sidewalk—left me out of breath and shaky. Falling asleep never came easily, and waking up in the morning was only successful when there was the promise of coffee within ten minutes of rising, and consistent subsequent cups throughout the day.

I worked hard and ate hard, and my body rebelled against me. I developed acne (which no medication would cure, and I tried them all), painful boils on my thighs where they constantly rubbed together, and even occasional abscesses in my ears. My eyes were in a constant state of puffiness, my mind in a constant state of fixation on when and where my next meal or coffee would be.

Yet, ironically, I was wildly successful at my career and was regularly given way more credit than I deserved by people who were inspired by my advocacy efforts, by the articles I wrote, by the talks I delivered. They grasped at anything they could find as a sign of hope for animal rights, which often seemed like such a hopeless cause that so many people—even otherwise decent, kind people— felt free to ignore. This kind of recognition humbled and jarred me, and all I could do to deal with it was to work even harder.

I was regularly giving workshops on veganism and on effective grassroots advocacy at festivals, universities, bookstores, and events throughout the country. Though I received countless e-mails following these presentations—most of which blend together for me—I can still recall with painful precision the ones (and there were a lot of them) that read something like "I just so admire your unabashed ability to get up there, despite your size," or, "The fact that you're comfortable with your body, even though you're large, is inspiring. There aren't enough fat women out there who will go to the microphone and be seen. Good for you."

Good for me? What, exactly, had I been doing that was so admirable? Not apologizing publicly for my fatness? Being an outspoken advocate even though my weight dictated that I should probably just shut up and be quiet, because opinions were for thin, beautiful women?

These comments, which were no doubt intended as compliments, made me incredibly uncomfortable. Even though I understood, on some level, that I was fat, I got through the majority of my days by pretending I wasn't. Similarly, even though I knew, on some level, that my physical ailments—the achiness, the headaches, the sore feet, the bad back—were a direct extension of my weight and my diet's lack of healthful foods, I convinced myself that it was just because I worked so hard.

What I lacked, clearly, was balance. But, as I said on an all-too-regular basis, *who needed balance* when there was a new vegan ice cream shop in the East Village?

It was, after all, for the animals.

THIRTEEN

—

that alone wasn't enough

Food was not the only love in my life.

There is a fine line between the way we relate to sex and the way we relate to food. For me, both were fraught with unfortunate choices, immense pleasure from sometimes surprising sources, obsessive desire, and—ultimately—nourishment and sweetness. Just as with food, I approached my romantic relationships with a fervor and fury that took over everything. My loves, whether of people or sugar, were not always the best choices for me, but—for better or worse—they were my sustenance. And the lack of awareness regarding the way I related to food was alarmingly similar to the way I related to my own sexuality.

It started, of course, with Timmy, the light-haired, sparkly eyed beauty who swept me off my feet during our summer stock adventure back in 1997. I was just shy of eighteen and had no idea that this summer romance would become a defining relationship for me, the one I would always look back on with a mix of longing, bittersweet affection, and eye rolling. It could certainly be argued that my attitude toward food during that formative time could be thought of symbolically as a metaphor for my willingness (or lack thereof, really) to look inside myself with honesty. I ate and ate and ate and ate, yet I never had enough. Though it would be years before I would recognize my unending hunger as something much deeper than simply a food craving—as a profound imbalance between my vision of myself and of the world—with Timmy, the similarities (at least in retrospect) were startling. I was constantly in search of *more* with him, certainly because my evolving needs were not being met in my relationship—and so my hunger, with Timmy, too, was insatiable. We did love each other—I *still* love Timmy—but we were ultimately incapable of growing together anymore (or at least unwilling to put in the work that kind of fortitude required), and, concurrently, we were completely unable to break things off.

One minute it was, "Jazz, I don't know what I'd do without you in my life . . ." which I responded to with a twenty-minute embrace and echoes of intense neediness. The next moment we were crying and physically pushing each other away, saying, "I don't want you anymore . . . I feel so trapped. Get out of my life!"

We loved and hated, fought and fucked. The emotional roller coaster of our relationship was inexplicable and based simply on habit and codependence. We had become adults together, and separating ourselves from those formative years seemed impossible, so we stayed together, each intensely focused on the other, despite our insurmountable differences. Though I think that strong relationships are those in which people can evolve together, and can inform each other's growth and even complement each other's weaknesses with one's own strengths, Timmy and I simply outgrew each other. We were too young (or immature) to commit to being in it with each other for the long run.

Still, there was that one special place we always managed to see eye to eye: food. The two of us became well practiced in taking late-night excursions to diners for eggs and toast, or to Dunkin' Donuts for two Boston creams each. We bonded over fried things, and as we ate them, they ate us—swallowing our relationship whole.

Food began to overshadow everything for us. It was like a tidal wave, soaking and rearranging everything in its path—even those parts of us that had otherwise been intact. Timmy, for example, had always been an avid runner and passionate motocross racer. But by the time I was twenty-one and he twenty-nine—by the time the tidal wave had started to rise—he'd traded in his athleticism for an early-onset beer gut. And as time passed, we, as a pair, seriously lost sight of our health (our go-to snack was a family-sized bag of Doritos each), and we dealt with our ultimate incompatibility by stuffing our faces so that our mouths were busy. If we couldn't talk, we couldn't break up, even though breaking up was clearly what we should've done. Although Timmy and I loved each other deeply, we were mutually destructive. We enabled one another, and—frighteningly—we also acted as a frame of reference: As Timmy gained weight, you couldn't really tell if I was gaining it, because I was still the same proportion to him. It was simple physics.

Looking back, I realize there was perhaps a more substantial reason behind our foray into food. The fact that I was a lesbian, but didn't know it yet, might have had something to do with the inconsistent sex and the emotional tumultuousness of our love affair. I loved him, and he loved me, but that alone wasn't enough.

Our five-year relationship was therefore not surprisingly an on-again, off-again affair, with the first "off" period being when I first went to college. While we eventually reconvened, there was one other off period—this one significant for other reasons. I was barely twenty at the time, and during this particular break from Timmy, I ventured into two new territories: AOL and lesbianism—or, as I defined it for myself at the time, bisexuality.

It wasn't as though I had been closeted before then—not to my knowledge, anyway. I realize that for many people, their sexual preference is strong from the moment they discover they're sexual beings, or perhaps even earlier. For me, growing up, my fascination with women was indeed intense, but I did not think of it as sexual attraction. However, my obsession with Bette Midler, and later, the Broadway star Patti LuPone, did seem to be a bit more than your run-of-the-mill aspiring actress's admiration. I absolutely adored them, and had an unwavering desire to be the most important person in their lives, but that brand of lust never felt salacious to me.

Perhaps more telling was my obsession with my young, female teachers—who, in retrospect, I was clearly crushing on (the roots of my later propensity toward teacher types, perhaps?). Many of my female teachers were deeply sexy to me, and I thought of them in the same ways I imagine many of the hormone-laden boys in my classes did. But, again, it never quite registered that these feelings were sexual, especially since I concurrently had crushes on boys (though I never felt for them nearly as much as I did for those glorious teachers).

Gay was something that happened to your cousin, not to you.

Gay was something you were "cool with," not something you embraced—certainly not on a personal level. To even entertain that thought felt fake, because clearly my trajectory was to get married to a man and have children. That was what I always assumed would happen, and that was what my mother and grand-mother assumed for me, too. It was simply never questioned, and there were no telltale signs I was gay—which was validated by the fact that I went through my early and midteen years writing bad poetry about not having a boyfriend, or dramatic, fictional-ized accounts of broken hearts.

Still, even if I didn't recognize them as such, I see now that there were indeed signs. Emily—the girl I met at the University of the Arts, who had inspired my initial vegetarianism—was the first lesbian I was friends with, and when we'd hang out, I was intensely aware of her sexual identity. When I'd spend time with one of my many gay male friends, I never even thought about their sexual preference, but there was something about sharing my space with gay women that made me feel extremely vulner-able, in ways I didn't understand and, perhaps, preferred not to think about.

Then, when I moved to New York and met Clara—the petite, spiral-haired rabble-rouser who held my hand when I stood up at *The Vagina Monologues*, my mind started to shift, just a little. On one particularly sunny day, when I was meeting Clara after the LGBT club meeting she was leading, I arrived early and waited outside. Clara spotted me through the window and made a simple, friendly gesture for me to join them. Upon seeing her invitation, my stomach was instantly in knots, my legs frozen beneath me. I shook my head no and, once my legs started working again, I feverishly walked away, wondering the whole time why I was reacting so strongly.

At night, I would lie awake and wonder why I was always so repulsed when men would reach orgasm. I realize how obvious all this sounds in retrospect, but when I was living through it, the dots never once connected. My plan was to get married to a man and have children. I was madly in love with Timmy and felt lucky to have discovered true love so early. Being a lesbian was something I was so, so far from ready for that I didn't even let my mind go there.

Until, that is, my mind went there.

When I started college, the Internet was just beginning to seep its way into mainstream culture. My first roommate had e-mail— I did not yet—and when she wasn't home, I would take the opportunity to jump on her computer and read Broadway forums; I created a screen name ("JazzPatti") and weighed in on how outraged I was that Patti LuPone did not get a Tony (embarrassingly, this is still Googleable). By the time I transferred to Pace University, I had my very own monster-sized computer, complete with my own e-mail address, courtesy of America Online. AOL was like a whole new world. Not only could I search for endless facts about Patti LuPone for hours on end, but, lit by the late-night glimmer of the computer screen, and put at ease by the newfound anonymity that the Internet effortlessly provided, I could dip my toe into lesbianism simply by clicking "women seeking women."

And that was how I met Natalie—a twenty-nine-year-old actress who lived in Queens—by a simple *click click click*.

"I've never done this before," I told her when we met for coffee at a tiny Chelsea café, which, itself, could have used a bit more anonymity. I noticed that my hand was shaking, and I don't think it was the caffeine.

"I've done enough for both of us," she said, with a wink, and no shaking whatsoever. With that, I was on the N train beside her, heading to Astoria, Queens, with nothing more than a Metro-Card and a relentless curiosity.

Natalie was obese—much heavier than I was—and I found an odd (and inappropriate) solace in my relative size to her. *I was the small one.* Our proportionality also made me feel she was easier to reach than, say, Clara, who was so thin, and clearly wouldn't be interested in someone my size.

At Natalie's apartment, which she shared with two other aspiring actors, we held hands and then leaned in for a kiss—my first with a woman, aside from the time I had to kiss one in my scene study class, which always caused me to break down laughing just before our faces met. I was truly shocked by how soft Natalie's lips were, as compared to the rough kisses and scruffy chins of the men I'd been with. Something about the kiss felt right (making me momentarily wonder, had all my previous kisses been wrong?) and managed to fall into place perfectly, like a puzzle with all the pieces that effortlessly gets finished.

I was so intrigued by sex with her—mostly because she was a *her*—but the truth is the sex itself was awkward and, much to my disappointment, unsatisfying. She was indeed "well-spoken" in the sex area, but we didn't fit as I had hoped we would. Perhaps my initial intrigue had more to do with her gender, and the inherently titillating nature of vaguely anonymous Internet sex, than with Natalie herself. I fumbled around with her, and she was charmingly patient. Of course, I'm sure many sexually active twenty-year-olds find that kind of intimacy awkward. I had spent so many years either ignoring, loathing, or abusing my body, how could I possibly share it in full with a veritable stranger? It's completely unsurprising, therefore, that I was just not feeling the sex with Natalie, even though I wanted so badly to see fireworks.

Unfortunately, that colossal disappointment subsequently kept me from following my urges to sleep with another woman again for many years. Naturally, it made me question my initial foray into lesbianism, and kept me from going back there—in full—for a long time. Throughout those years, I did indeed fool around with quite a few women anyway—but with our clothes (mostly) on. When it came to making out with them, I always managed to stop things just before they switched into full gear—afraid I wouldn't like it again, or maybe afraid I'd like it too much.

The person who finally did me in—the last remaining ingredient in my embracing my lesbianism—was Denise, a butch woman eighteen years older than me, and about as wonderfully feminist as you can get. I was instantly enamored with her. Hearkening back to my relationship with Timmy, and, really, to my adolescent relationship with Burger King, my crush quickly became obsession. She was a professor, a writer, a brainy academic, and a brooding artist. She was also vegan, a committed animal activist, and my newest fanatical focus.

Everything I did became colored by what I thought Denise would think. I wanted to embody her passionate dedication to living ethically—I was in love with her commitment and, I thought, in love with her as well. As a result, I forgot myself somewhere.

After spending months communicating through phone calls that ostensibly regarded an article I was interviewing her for—calls that often expanded into discussions about life and all its meanings—it didn't take long for me to get over my fear of sex when we finally met in person for the first time. Specifically, it took about two hours from when we met. And even though I was enamored with her brain, it was sex with Denise that truly blew my mind. With men, I had constantly been self-conscious—always leaving my shirt on so that they couldn't see my enormous stomach, which I was certain would make them run away, midthrust. But Denise not only didn't mind my curves, she celebrated them. Sex with her was the first time I ever knew what it meant to surrender completely to the natural rhythms of your own body, and your partner's. It was after one of these lusty encounters that Denise looked at me, half smiled, and quietly proclaimed with her raspy, deep voice, "I totally think you're a lesbian."

And that was that.

As part of my intense longing for her (*all things Denise, all the time*), I began to notice the way she ate, and—seeing everything she did as emblematic of her fierce feminism—I tried to replicate that, too.

One day, as she sat in her study working, I decided to make lunch. Pretty much the only things in her fridge were white bread, vegan mayo, and vegan bologna. I stared at the bologna and I was eight years old again, in the bathroom stall during lunch, shutting out the sadness and escaping into the familiar reassurance of my food.

Usually, that would have been the moment when I would have fought with myself about whether it would be a wise move to eat that sandwich. I would hem and haw, ruminating and rationalizing—and eventually would wind up eating it anyway, though with immense regret.

But, hold on—*Denise did it*. She ate white bread with vegan bologna and didn't even feel bad about it. So surely the *feminist* thing to do would be to eat the bologna sandwich, and stop with this asinine desire to please other people by conforming my body to what society thought it should look like.

Illuminated by both the fridge light and the simple, but startling revelation that feverishly exploded inside of me, I decided then and there to not give a damn anymore about getting fat(ter). I decided to try life sans the self-imposed guilt, and with a heaping side of vegan mayo. I would *devour* that dazzling sandwich.

Sadly, Denise got over me almost as quickly as she got her gold star for bringing me out of the closet in full. My heart was shattered—so much of my identity had inexplicably (and inappropriately) been wrapped up in her.

I was living in Washington Heights at the time, in the northernmost part of Manhattan. After our breakup (though I'd venture to guess Denise didn't see it as a breakup, since she probably never considered it a relationship in the first place), a friend of mine, Sara, insisted on taking me out for a drink. We sat there eating fries and drinking red wine. "I just don't know who I am anymore," I told Sara. "I don't know what I like."

Sara thought about this, then offered, "You like purple eye shadow, Jazz. Why don't you start with that?"

It sounds so minor—beginning the process of reclaiming yourself with the simple power of eye makeup. And yet Sara's suggestion touched me, and stuck with me. I had allowed Denise's presence to replace my identity, my purple eye shadow. I had indeed lost my color. Only when I began to reapply it did I start to reapply myself to my life.

"I am giving you an ultimatum," I said to Mariann, who had made the bold and adorable choice to wear overalls. We were sitting at House of Vegetarian in Chinatown—the only two people in the restaurant. Outside, a midafternoon summertime thunderstorm blanketed the city. The sky was a grayish pink and dotted with bright flecks of lightning.

We had, as usual, ordered enough food for all of lower Manhattan to feast on. Embarrassingly, the waiter pushed together two more small tables so that we could easily reach our dim sum selections, including her favorite and mine: fried turnip cakes.

"You're *huh*?" asked Mariann, as she stole a steamed dumpling with her chopsticks.

"I'm presenting you with an ultimatum," I repeated, nervously fiddling with the letter I'd written her earlier that day—the letter proclaiming that if we couldn't be more than friends, then I couldn't continue to know her.

Suddenly channeling my inner seventh grader, I quickly handed Mariann my note and awkwardly excused myself to go to the bathroom.

Ever since my friend Marisa had married Mariann's friend David the previous May (not the tuna-eating David from the park), she and I had spoken every day. Somewhere around our third dance at the wedding reception, I had officially become smitten with her, and I was intent on not letting her get away. Our friendship quickly became powerful and intimate, consisting of shared watermelon slices and tearful confessions about the pain we'd each felt as outsiders looking in.

Always deeply sensitive—not to mention a grade-A introvert—Mariann had simply been one of those people who never felt she quite belonged, despite the world treating her as if she did. She was, I later found out, a closeted outsider, playing the part as best she could so that no one would notice. Mariann had also been single for most of her life, choosing to spend the majority of her time with her dogs as opposed to with lovers. Her propensity toward being unpartnered in a society that celebrates coupledom and inexplicably looks down at the single life, combined with her long-time veganism (she was vegan long before veganism was ever a headline in the *New York Times*), had sufficiently acclimated her to the feeling of going up the down staircase. Perhaps life was most efficiently tackled when alone—or, rather, with the help of trusted canines and their unconditional love. The fact that she began to let me in, when so few others had been allowed there, was flattering, but also it allowed me the great privilege of loving the parts of her that made her the most special, unique, and insightful human being I had ever known. Lucky, lucky me.

By the time we connected, we also had each recently been involved in a nasty breakup—one of Mariann's few, and her first with a woman. (She describes herself as a "late-breaking lesbian.") So, in addition to a shared worldview, the two of us bonded over our broken hearts and our popped bubbles. Mariann was patient, empathic, and encouraging—traits I had longed for in a partner. She was also deeply sexy—the kind of "buttoned-up professor" that I loved to unbutton.

Prior to that day in Chinatown, I had already known that I loved Mariann intensely, and yet—as I stood in the bathroom stall counting to a hundred—I was well aware that when I returned to the table, she would immediately bring up the eight-hundred-pound gorilla as the reason we couldn't be more than friends. And for once, it wasn't my size.

Mariann is twenty-nine and a half years older than me. I was not yet twenty-eight, and she was fifty-seven.

I remember talking to a therapist once about my fascination

with older women—teacher types, mostly—wondering aloud if it was a personality flaw, a weird fetish in which I should not indulge. He looked at me, shrugged, and in one simple sentence he let me off the hook. "Maybe . . . that's just your type?" I digested that distinct possibility—which I'd never before considered—and returned his nonchalant shrug.

It's astonishing how easily we sometimes classify our personality traits as *flaws*, obsessing about them unnecessarily—and it's just as amazing how even just the tiniest validation and perspective can bring us back to earth. (Two points for therapy.)

Still in the bathroom at Vegetarian Dim Sum, I kept counting, willing away my butterflies. *Forty-nine . . . fifty . . . fifty-one . . . Maybe she'll surprise me . . .*

I glanced at myself in the mirror. It occurred to me that since Mariann had entered my life, I somehow saw myself differently. I was, you might argue, just a little bit lovely looking—if you cocked your head just right. And squinted your eyes.

Ninety . . . ninety-one . . . ninety-two . . .

Wait—did I really just look at myself and think *lovely*? What was this otherworldly power that this woman—this *truly* beautiful woman—had over my attitude? Was she seriously dismantling my cynical, jaded exterior? How was it that, after a lifetime of feeling *less than*—and of being treated as such—I was finally beginning to feel grounded, even just a little bit?

Surely Mariann must love me back.

Sadly, my hunch that she'd be a tough sell was correct. Returning to the table, I noticed—despite the flyaway bangs that partially covered her gigantic blue eyes—that she was teary. "This is the nicest thing anyone has ever given to me," she told me, as I sank further and further into my chair and into my longing. "But if you force me to choose, I'm going to say no. It's not that I don't care. You know I do. In many ways I feel closer to you than I've ever felt to anyone. But I can't handle the age difference. It just doesn't work."

And just at that moment, the lightning outside struck my heart and I was both scared and scheming, trying desperately hard to get out of this pickle I'd gotten myself into—because, my God, I could not live my life without this woman.

So I reneged, telling her that by *ultimatum* I really meant *possibility*, and, sure, let's still be friends. Let's still hang out and listen to old records together. Let's make important life decisions two by two, as *chums*. Let's call each other when our cats die or our nieces are born. Or, hell, let's just call each other every night. But let's pretty please not be out of each other's lives.

The rain was unrelenting, and twenty minutes after I accepted my Olympic medal for *backpedaling*, and as we walked toward her tiny apartment in Soho, we let it soak through our clothes and our spirits. On Prince Street near West Broadway, I suddenly stopped walking, and then Mariann did, too. I pulled her into me, and we stood like that for ten minutes, crying along with the sky.

Two weeks later, as we stood on another street corner—this time in Midtown, where I was heading off to rehearse for a play— Mariann kissed me. It was only half on the mouth, but it was a clear and conscious proclamation. *We will love each other differently now*, the kiss said, and we did just that.

Our age difference became a nonissue, and our shared worldview became our bottom line. We loved together, laughed together, and ate together. We plotted together, created together, and healed together. We held each other when we couldn't sleep, and held on to each other when the world became too much.

And when I would weep because I wanted to rip my body off

of myself—they were, after all, two separate entities, my body and my self—Mariann would call me beautiful. When I would grab my stomach by the fistful and scream, Mariann would call me luscious. And when the world treated me unfairly, Mariann would see in me not the lost soul I felt I was at that moment, but the extraordinary person who, against all my expectations, she was sure that I was, and would continue to become.

Many years before, as I sat on the stage in my high school, in the bright and unforgiving spotlight, and I heard the laughter in the audience—when my scene partner coldly looked away, afraid my fatness could possibly be contagious—I remember firmly believing that my life would very likely be lived alone. I had spent years since then trying to prove myself wrong; trying by way of my ultimately unsuccessful relationship with Timmy, then with subsequent fleeting and failed dalliances with many other women and men. Each and every time, those very flings left me feeling lonelier than I had before them, and the gaping hole in my heart constantly became deeper. But when Mariann adamantly kept her gaze on me, refusing to look away—even when I tested her by showing her my ugliest parts—I finally relented. I decided to trust in the reflection I saw when I looked at myself through her eyes. Mariann loved me. I was lovable. I was *loved*.

And so why not love myself a little, too?

We were in it together, she and I. We were connected in ways we didn't—and might never—fully understand.

And so Mariann and I became a couple, fused at the hip and at the heartstrings. I moved into that tiny apartment in Soho, and her gorgeous pit bull Rose became my sweet dog, too. I settled gracefully into my new life in lower Manhattan, with my dog and my partner beside me, and my heart swollen with goodness inside me.

And yet, despite the serenity I finally found, food remained firmly my enemy. Even though my heart was finally full, my stomach refused to be. I ate more and more food, more feverishly than I had before, and I got bigger as Mariann got bigger, too—right alongside me, where she always was.

Habit is perhaps the strongest force there is—stronger sometimes than resolve, stronger often than knowledge. Even the greatest love cannot override the most deeply instilled habit. Even the sweet reflection of yourself as seen through your doting partner's eyes cannot stand a chance next to the sweetness of a cupcake, when that cupcake is all you have ever known.

And then, one day, that very habit formed a tiny but unmistakable crack down the middle. In the wake of a fateful falafel-filled night in San Francisco, Mariann and I made a simple, but somehow intrepid decision to start a juice fast together. And our world became an ultimatum: Either live truthfully, and reclaim our health, or fail, knowing that we did our best, and our best just wasn't enough.

III

what i changed

FOURTEEN

we'll see what happens [days 1–5]

On September 1, 2010, shortly after getting back from San Francisco, Mariann and I started our first ten-day juice fast. I documented the whole thing, daily, in a "vlog" on YouTube, and on the first day I said to Mariann, "I'm aiming for ten days. We'll see what happens."

What happened was that I indeed finished those ten days, as did Mariann. What happened was I lost eleven pounds in those ten days. What happened was I spent those ten days schooling myself on the healing power of vegetables and whole foods. What happened was Mariann wound up walking to her office with a huge rolling suitcase full to bursting with compostable food scraps, to drop off at the compost container in Union Square. What happened was I gave up coffee, cold. What happened was we committed to doing another juice fast the following month—for three days—and planned for another ten-day fast for the month after that.

Thus began the trajectory of the next three years of our lives.

We juiced each month: ten days one month, three days the following, then ten, then three, and so on. We juiced in the sweltering summers when the pavement in Manhattan was literally steaming, and we juiced in the bitterly cold winters when the city was blanketed with an unrelenting deep snow. Within two years of starting my first juice fast, I was down nearly one hundred pounds, where I have remained—it is my new normal.

But before it was normal, it was terrifying. I suppose the same thing can be said about anything life changing that you do for the first time—from driving to sex to moving out on your own to moving into middle age. Everything requires getting used to, and some things, more than others, have a steep learning curve. When your life is governed by your relationship to food—and most of ours are, at least to some extent—and then, kind of overnight, you completely change the way you consume, your world inevitably shifts. And when your life is defined by your size, as mine was, undergoing a drastic change such as losing nearly one hundred pounds dramatically affects the way you see the world, the way the world sees you, and just about everything in between.

Since I had first been turned on to juicing, thanks to the documentary *Fat, Sick & Nearly Dead* by Joe Cross, my juicing commenced by largely following the program Joe recommended. When I first started, I drank five juices a day, beginning with a fruit juice such as apple/ginger or orange/grapefruit, with all the other juices throughout the day heavily revolving around greens, with some fruit (such as a couple of apples or pears) mixed in for a touch of sweetness. I was also having water with lemon in between juices.

The juices were large—each one filled up a giant mason jar—and inexplicably filling. My biggest fear of juicing, of course, was that I would be hungry. For my entire life, the idea of hunger had petrified me. Hunger meant weakness, scarcity, and longing. Hunger also allowed in the painful feelings that I so conveniently could abolish with food; when the going got rough, I got lunch. It petrified me to think that I would be experiencing hunger and not be able to treat it.

Years later, in 2013, during the months, weeks, and days just before my grandma died, a therapist I was seeing referred to my extreme emotional turmoil as "anticipatory grief." In some ways, that period was worse than the actual grief that followed Grandma's death. Perhaps the fear of hunger with which I was so obsessed before starting my juice fast could be called "anticipatory hunger."

However, unlike my fear of the grief to come when Grandma was dying, my fear as I anticipated the hunger to come as I started my first juice fast was unfounded. In fact, and I know this sounds unlikely, it turned out that once I got used to juice fasting, I wasn't very hungry at all. And so the anticipatory fear was a waste of energy.

I remember in some detail my first ten-day juice fast—from September 1 through September 10, 2010, because I video documented it. So let me break it down for you.

day 1

The first juicer I used I found under a quarter inch of dust in the back of our very own kitchen cupboard. It was an antiquated Jack LaLanne model that Mariann had bought in the 1990s. I'm almost certain that the first juice I consumed included a healthy dose of that dust, since I coughed my way through it. Either that or my body was in shock at the introduction of fruits and vegetables.

Incidentally, the second juicer I got—only the following month—was another "lightly used" model, and the way I picked it up resembled a drug deal. A random Facebook "friend"—who I had never met before, and was only connected with in cyberland because of our shared interest in animal rights—offered it to me when my status update whined about my very privileged problem of my juices having "too much pulp and not enough liquid!!!" Turned out this Good Samaritan was in the middle of downsizing and was grateful to pass on her used machine to a juicer-in-need. We made the transfer at Grand Central Station on a Tuesday during the afternoon rush hour. I had agreed to pay for her train ticket back to Connecticut, so, when we spotted one another at the right place and time, she slipped me the machine and I covertly handed her a white envelope. Then we nodded and quickly went off on our own way, me with yet another antiquated juicer in hand, which I could barely lift—and which, it turned out, could barely produce juice.

When I look back on the early days of my juicing, one thought trumps all others: *What the hell was I thinking?*

On day one of my very first fast, my thoughts went something like this: "I'm hungry, my stomach hurts, and I'm a little nauseous—though I'm still determined to get through this."

With my Jack LaLanne doing its very best, I started off the day with apple juice with some kale and ginger. "Can't get enough ginger," I said in my video log (now when I listen to it, I wonder if I actually hear a bit of sarcasm). At eleven A.M., I had a green juice with kale, spinach, parsley, cucumber, an apple, lemon, and, of course, loads of ginger. The greens' taste was offset a bit by the apple, ginger, and lemon, but barely enough to make the juice palatable. Despite the juice's bitterness, it tasted surprisingly decent, and I remember thinking that it would be even better with a shot of vodka.

At the same time, despite my own bitterness, I nonetheless felt I was flooding my body with nutrients, and somehow that seemed to compensate for the mildly bitter aftertaste of the juice-meal. Sadly, an hour later, I started to get hungry and almost crashed when I accidentally saw a picture of a plate of brownies on my Facebook feed (thankfully, prior to the juice fast, we had purged our fridge and cabinets of anything tempting, or edible for that matter). Instead of giving in to the momentary temptation (the very stocked corner bodega was only a half block away), I forced myself to shut the computer off and I kept going, knowing that my next juice was only an hour away.

"It's always hard when you're beginning something like this because you kind of always want to know how it's going to turn out," I said to the camera. I wish I had known how it would, in fact, turn out. Had I realized just what a life-altering role juice would play in my life—with results of my efforts showing just days into my first fast—I would have perhaps had a healthier attitude, so to speak. When I started juicing, I was skeptical. If I had only known how successful the endeavor would ultimately be, I wonder if I would have been a bit more of a trouper, at least while consuming the yuckier of the juices. During those early days, though I had high hopes, I thought there was no way that I would be able to predict even a fraction of the outcome—the outcome being that my decision to go on a juice fast would indeed change the course of my life.

Even from that first day, I recognized how lucky I was to be doing this with Mariann. Having someone to share it with was deeply helpful. I didn't want to let myself down, and I didn't want to let her down, either. And I knew she felt the same way. And we both knew that, if one of us slipped, the other was much more likely to as well. Sometimes doing something for someone you love—especially something that is helping to make them healthier—is easier than doing it solely for yourself. Also, having someone else in the house who was abstaining from eating real food was a blessing. Anyone doing a juice fast needs to find some sort of support, even if it is online, and could use as much cooperation as possible from anyone in the house who isn't joining in. The last thing anyone needs during a juice fast is a chocolate-mouthed spouse or kid tempting them with cake or fries. (Though I suppose a good retort would be to threaten them that if they don't cut it out, they'll be forced to sample the juices that have mustard greens—which I have found consistently taste like running shoes. Not that I've ever tasted my running shoes.)

In the middle of that first day, Mariann, who was at her office (I worked from home), called and said she was exhausted and kept nodding off at her desk. While my worst symptom was cravings, and Mariann's was lethargy, my guess is that they were both attributable to the same cause—i.e., to the fact that we each had so much crap to detox. These days when we juice fast, though there is still some degree of tiredness and hunger, it's not anything notable. Perhaps that's because our bodies began to know what to expect, but it's more likely a result of the fact that all the toxins we needed to detox that first time—toxins left over from a diet heavy in caffeine, sugar, processed foods—are no longer at the center of our nonjuicing diets, so the detox isn't as big for us now. For people who consume animal products, the detox process would no doubt be even more intense and, likely, the symptoms of detox more harrowing. The crappier your diet—in other words, the further away it is from whole foods—the more painful the initial detox.

But cravings still occur, and I should know. It seems the Facebook images of brownies had seeped their way into my consciousness, because I started to see little brownies parading around in my mind's eye like a group of protesters, begging for my attention. Old habits die hard, and cravings can destroy your best intentions. Even these days when I juice fast, I try hard to limit my access to triggering images, like pictures of my friends' yummy dinners and desserts on social media (vegans love to post photos of their meals). The destroyer of many of my lifelong plans to fight food cravings, those dreaded TV commercials (I have a soft spot for the Pop-Tart ads, and don't even put me in the same room as a waffle commercial), are not as much of an issue since my TV watching has mostly shifted to online, but for many of us there are still images of food everywhere we look. Regardless of whether I would actually give in to the cravings that visual imagery can provoke, it's an additional complication and frustration that I can easily avoid.

I had read that it was important, especially for our first juice fast, for Mariann and me to get our bodies ready for it by spending a few days beforehand consuming whole foods and slowing or stopping the consumption of coffee, alcohol, sugar, and highly processed foods. We planned to do the same thing afterward, as we reacclimated ourselves to food. It would make the process that much more difficult if we were jumping into this juice fast with a hangover, for example, or a rabid coffee addiction. Mariann and I needed to give our bodies a few days on either end to make the process easier, and to allow ourselves a chance to adjust, physically and emotionally, to consuming only juice. Though I was by no means perfect in this, in the days leading up to day one, I made a conscious effort to up my intake of vegetables and to eat fewer sweets. (Admittedly, however, the final meal I had the night before day one was two slices of vegan cheesecake, my very favorite kind from Teany on the Lower East Side.) In an ideal world, I wouldn't have eaten any junk food in those days leading up to day one, but until the juicer grumbled and spit for the first time on that first day, I simply wasn't all in. Once I was, however, I was committed to giving this juicing thing a serious go.

day 2

On the positive side, I had a lot more energy than I thought I would, but on the negative, I was overwhelmed at the thought that I was only on day two and had eight more days to go. I was hungry, of course, but the hunger still wasn't that bad, which completely amazed me.

My morning fruit juice was grapefruit, my absolute favorite. After that, I tried a more eclectic concoction of spinach, parsley, kale, cucumber, celery, ginger, peach, and apple.

As you may have guessed, since I was making all these juices, I was spending a lot of time slaving over the juicer (still the subpar Jack LaLanne at this point). One solution was that I tried to get the process of actually making the juice down to two or three times a day—in other words, I would make all of my and Mariann's five juices for the day in two or three sessions of juicing. Many juicing aficionados constantly reiterate the importance of consuming the juice as soon as possible after it is made (the immediacy of consuming it also depends on the type of juicer you're using), and though I tried my best to adhere to that rule, I also had to do what was realistic for me in my life—so I simply did the best I could. Creating the day's juices in two or three sittings was much more realistic for me, allowing me not to spend all my time juicing and cleaning the juicer.

I admit that I quickly became one of those people for whom juicing takes over their lives. When I wasn't drinking it, I was thinking about it; when I wasn't thinking about it, I was making it; and when I wasn't making it, I was drenching the entire kitchen counter and floor with water from cleaning the goddamn Jack LaLanne. It was big and clunky, and it didn't fit under our small Manhattan faucet with much dignity. I wonder now if perhaps the reason I lost weight during that first juice fast had something to do with the workout I was getting simply from spending so much time doing the dishes.

The other thing I was spending was money. Juice fasts—which may be more accurately called "juice cleanses" or "juice feasts" (if you want to be annoying, since you are actually consuming lots of food)—are "expensive as hell," as I said in my video log at the time, no doubt nervous at seeing how much produce I was going through already. At the time, I was wedded to doing it all organic, whenever possible. I tried not to think too much about the money—we had actually budgeted for the juice fast and, after all, it was reassuring to remember that we weren't going out to eat, or ordering in takeout, at all. (During a few of my weaker moments, I wondered if fried bean curd from my favorite Chinese place would fit in the juicer.)

Still, it was pricey. I could already see at this point that making any kind of long-term commitment to juicing would likely make a pretty big dent in our food budget. In fact, after the initial few juice fasts, my "rule" about consuming only organic juices began to bend a bit. I consulted the "Dirty Dozen" list, which is a list the Environmental Working Group puts together that spells out the fruits and vegetables that contain the most pesticides and are the most important to consume organically. The list varies a bit from year to year; when I last checked, it included apples, celery, cherry tomatoes, cucumbers, grapes, hot peppers, nectarines (imported), peaches, potatoes, spinach, strawberries, and sweet bell peppers—with kale, collard greens, and summer squash running close behind. Whenever I could, I continued to buy those items organic.

But for the other fruits and vegetables that weren't on the list, I used a high-quality fruit and vegetable scrub and then didn't worry so much about whether they were organic, which helped financially. It also helped in cutting down on the amount of time I was investing in juicing. We were going through a ton of produce, and even taking the time to go to the store and purchase it became exhausting. We were lucky in that we had a small, twenty-four-hour grocery store with ample produce a half block from our apartment. But organic produce was simply not always an option, and so my initial guidelines for *all organic, all the time* eventually began to bend.

As for physical reactions, I felt as though my lymph nodes—particularly the ones on the back of my head near the top of my neck—were a little swollen. (This has been true throughout my life; whenever I am under the weather, the two lymph nodes on the back of my head become gigantic—like two gumballs.) Mariann, on the other hand, experienced a bit of heartburn in those first few days of juicing; I did not. That's because her body goes there during detox. Detox tends to temporarily magnify the symptoms each of us has always experienced when our bodies go out of whack.

Maybe I sound like a masochist, voluntarily forcing my body to experience symptoms that, for most of my life, I have done my best to avoid. If you look at it as a short-term process, that may be true, but, in the long term, until I detoxed from the harmful foods I had been feeding it my whole life, I was not able to heal—not only physically, but mentally.

In fact, one of the most important things I eventually learned to look forward to when I juiced was the ability to give my brain a rest from thinking about food. This kind of "mental detox" was unexpected, but it evolved to become my cornerstone. It sounds counterintuitive to say that dedicating ten days to juicing—planning for it, making it, drinking it—allowed me room to focus on things that aren't food related, since in some ways it is *all* about food. But for me, the formula of having five juices a day (which eventually evolved to become six) actually freed my brain from worrying about where my next meal (or coffee) was going to come from. It allowed me to focus on rebooting my system and starting fresh—free of the mental and physical triggers that normally caused me to simply run to the cabinet for the Oreos.

day 3

This was the worst day so far. I was way more wonky than on days one and two, and, while I was anticipating that it would get easier after day three, I not only made a juice that was truly repulsive (it happens—especially when you combine collard greens with celery, kale, and garlic), but I received some feedback from some Facebook friends who thought what I was doing was "extreme," and I had to work to not let that get to me. I reminded myself, "Though it sounds really extreme, I think it's a very natural part of healing your own body and your own self."

I was also trying to find support online, and not just criticism. I read an interview with someone who had done a whopping ninety-day juice fast and had relied on a Post-it on her fridge that read, *You can do this. You are cleaning every cell and organ in your body. The struggle is temporary. You will feel so much better!* I got over the image of Stuart Smalley looking in the mirror and telling himself, "I'm good enough, I'm strong enough, and doggone it, people like me!" and put that saying on my fridge as well, and that simple affirmation actually helped immeasurably.

I found that physically, I was sated from the juices—not extremely hungry by any means, and certainly energetic enough to go through my days with relative normalcy. The truly hard part was readjusting my brain not to deal with my anxiety, my boredom, and even just my longing for the happiness I experienced by way of eating, by mindlessly running to the fridge.

This kind of impulse and this brand of longing goes far beyond simply a physical addiction or craving. Like many people, I have always used food as a way to assuage feelings and, to be honest, I don't think there was necessarily anything wrong with that in and of itself. Food is one of the greatest joys in life, and there's no reason not to use it as a means of celebration, ritual, and even dealing with feelings. And there's no reason that using food as a way to help manage moods needs to be considered inherently a "bad thing." If a nice little snack in the middle of a wearing afternoon (or post-run pancakes, my drug of choice these days after particularly long runs) relaxes you and cheers you up, that's fantastic. We all need some cheer. There's no reason why food shouldn't be used as a means of comfort. It's part of the greatness of eating, and something that bonds everyone in the world together. Food is about ritual, about sharing, about celebrating, and about enjoying ourselves. But, for me, the use of food as therapy had, for most of my life, simply taken over and had become the primary way I dealt with my feelings (Pop-Tarts make excellent shrinks). That is a whole lot more likely to happen when the foods you're eating are highly addictive and nutrient deficient, which described my diet, in spades. And that was the story of my life, up until juice.

For me, when I juice fast—and this was especially true during that first time—I find that the thing I have to get used to the most is not eating my feelings, and not dealing with life's normal pitfalls solely by way of food. I have found, actually, that this break from the constant choice and availability of food, and the concurrent abundant consumption of nutrients, creates a wonderful opportunity for delving deeper into my psyche and allowing myself the room to heal the parts of me that haven't otherwise had that chance.

Prior to my juice fasting, it was simply understood that if I had a bad day, or a bad moment, I would run to the fridge for a spoonful of icing, or to the cabinet for a handful of pretzels (to be followed, of course, by several more handfuls). This is pretty common behavior for a lot of us. Food is our drug. Which is probably better than having actual drugs be our drug, in which case, simply replace "a handful of pretzels" with a quick fix of *fill-in-the-blank*.

But for my entire life, my personal relationship with food went so far beyond balance that it entered dangerous territory and became my lifelong shield against the world and against living my own truth. Food brilliantly and frighteningly kept me from facing everything I didn't want to face, from the more existential pain of recognizing the realities of living in an unjust world to the much more personal painful feelings associated with recognizing those areas where I needed to grow inside myself. Once I began to detox my body from things like sugar, I was able to begin the process of detoxing my mind and heart, too, and figure out why it was that I so mindlessly ran to the fridge for my fix. It wasn't until after I began the detox process that I was able to begin the process of truly embracing and accepting myself for the fabulous and flawed person I was. It all started with juice.

During that first juice fast, I wanted Oreos. I wanted cake. I wanted French fries. Admittedly, dreams crept in at night with Teany's vegan cheesesteak in the starring role. I would wake up drooling (which, okay, I usually did anyway . . .), lusting after the creamy desserts and savory meals I wanted to ravage. In the early days of juicing, these foods haunted my nights, and sometimes my daydreams, too. I remember once saying out loud, but meaning to only think it, "I want cake."

"Don't go there," Mariann responded, battling her own food fantasies.

I wanted cake, but what I had in front of me instead was kale juice with some ginger and apple. I knew that I had made that commitment to myself—*ten days or bust.* I would stick to it no matter what.

What happened was that instead of grabbing for the Oreos, I started to think of why I wanted them in the first place. Why were they so comfortable and familiar to me? Why were they so reliable? And, for that matter, what did it mean for me to rely on something else instead of cookies to get me through an anxious or fraught day?

I've read that many people find that meditation is helpful while juice fasting. I admit that I am not one of those people, because, though the intention has been there, I have never figured out a way to work traditional meditation into my life (which is probably reason enough to do it). Frankly, I'd rather stick a fork in my eye than meditate, especially during a juice fast (though at least I'd be putting a fork into *something*).

But even without traditional meditation, there are most certainly moments of my life that bring me that same kind of mental clarity and calmness, such as being out in nature, taking a walk, or—these days—going for a run by myself. Juice fasting creates an opening to bask in meditative moments—whatever they are for you. It makes the "break" from eating that much more conscious and intentional, giving you more bang for the buck. When followed through, it can jolt you into consciousness about your consumption—at least, it did for me.

Moving from the metaphysical to the practical, during that third day when I was struggling with some pretty deep emotions and a rich (pun intended) fantasy life, Mariann and I were developing a pretty severe garbage situation. Juicing leaves a lot of bulk behind, and it seemed a shame to just throw out all those beautiful remnants of organic produce. Our solution was to keep our compost in the freezer until we were able to drop it off at the Union Square compost bin. This is probably easier for people who aren't city dwellers and can compost on their own, or even city dwellers who live in places where compost is now picked up at the curb, but, alas, Manhattanites do not have those luxuries.

In any case, the waste produced from juicing, and the impetus to find the most ethically sound and responsible way of managing it, can clearly be looked at as one big fat metaphor. Feeding this so-called waste back to the planet through composting, and realizing that when it's reused in a new way with a new purpose, it can actually be beneficial and instigate growth, is a very healing thought. Perhaps my very own bundles of emotional waste could follow suit, be replanted, and wind up being useful, rather than simply being tossed aside.

day 4

Day four was better, but didn't improve things as much as I had hoped. In fact, my dog Rose's food (which *is* vegan) began to look a bit too appetizing. I was also tired, and a bit foggy brained, and decided to allow myself to lie down and rest every now and then. I took a bath, which was not only restful, but had the added benefit of helping with the detox.

I decided that it would help me understand what was happening, and help me on my journey, to do some reading on detoxing, food addiction, and juicing. I chose to start with *The Pleasure Trap* by Douglas Lisle and Alan Goldhamer, which focuses on our addiction to excess (food and otherwise) and offers solutions to unintentional self-sabotage. Reading that book started a tradition for Mariann and me and, to this day, when we juice fast, we make an effort to read, watch, and listen to something every day that informs our juicing and our subsequent food plan. This works as a combined minivacation and self-directed fast-track learning program. And, always, it helps to keep me on the juice.

This time, from my online reading and watching, I found out that, as healthy as green juices are, we needed to limit the amount of beet greens and red chard and, to some extent, spinach, because of the oxalic acid present in them, which can decrease calcium absorption and shouldn't be consumed in huge quantities. *Good to know.* I found it out the hard way, actually, by getting a scratchy throat that I later found out was due to consuming too much of that oxalic acid. Remaining conscious of how much of those particular greens I juiced was certainly no reason to cut down on other greens, though, since they are so good for you, and, in fact, four out of the five juices I consumed daily were greens based. We continued our practice of starting off the day with a fruit juice, though, and on day four it was watermelon juice, which thrilled me probably more than it should have.

day 5

Admittedly, I was tired. I was, in fact, very tired. I tried to convince myself that it was because I had exercised the previous day—for the first time in as long as I was able to remember.

Not too long before we embarked on this juicing journey, Mariann and I had invested in a Nintendo Wii Fit, which was perfect for me since I didn't have to go out of the house and be seen in order to exercise. There had been an intriguing article in the *New York Times* about the Wii Fit, and we were officially hooked by precisely what the program became famous for, the mix of playing games and burning calories. (Being a child of the eighties, I was also extremely excited about reintroducing Dr. Mario into my life.) But I was hardly in good shape, and a juice fast was probably the worst possible time for me to shock my system into exercising, especially given the fact that I was not used to it. I needed to remind myself that I didn't have as much energy as I usually did, and even if I did have energy, I'm sure that beginning an exercise regimen, given my usual sedentary ways, would be physically jarring.

A lot of what I had read about juice fasts talked about how

great people felt, especially after the third day. How much energy and vibrancy they experienced. So even though I was able to partially blame my fatigue on my need for instant gratification by way of my Wii Fit, it was a bit discouraging to find that I was still feeling tired.

And so, feeling discouraged and wanting to reenergize and motivate myself, I started examining my motives for doing the juice fast in the first place. I was deliberately not weighing myself regularly and I was quite adamant that I was not doing this cleanse to lose weight. (As an important side note, Wii Fit offered the option of getting weighed without displaying the number, so I did that, only checking back on the actual number much later— once I was able to stomach the truth.) Instead of regularly hopping onto the scale, I reported by way of my vlog that the juice fast was "a reboot, a way to get rid of some nasty addictions you might have, or nasty habits. And it's also really good emotionally, too." I stressed that "it allows you to slow down in your life and just take things a little bit more easy."

Detox. That was the name of the game, not weight loss. And, throughout any detox process, some negative symptoms are inevitable. Even somebody who doesn't have weight to lose could still benefit from doing a juice fast because of its detoxifying properties, both physically and mentally.

Thinking of the juice fast as motivated by detox, rather than weight loss, helped me in other ways beyond just helping me to explain and tolerate my negative symptoms. Juicing with the mind-set of doing it for health, rather than doing it for weight loss per se, really shifted things for me and allowed me to come at it from a much more open and less defensive, place.

And the incentives were powerful. The fact that I had high

triglycerides, which my doctor had made clear at my recent physical, meant I was on my way to heart disease. Plus there was the
fact that I was constantly fatigued. During that first juice fast,
there were times when even just carrying my weight around felt
taxing. "I'm going to stand up now," I would say to Mariann,
who—from her seated position across the room—would say,
"Okay, honey . . . I know you can do it."

"I'm going to . . ." I would respond, still sitting there.

"Good," she'd say.

"But first I'm going to rest."

"Sounds like a plan," Mariann would respond, supportively.

A few minutes later, I'd stand up, overdramatically grunting
the whole way, for effect.

Perhaps my fatigue was partially caused by an emotional
weight, too. I started to see my detox symptoms—swollen lymph
nodes, mild tiredness, and hunger—as something I just had to get
through in order to heal and become healthy, even if that meant
confronting what lay beneath, the reasons I had so eagerly opted
for instant gratification in the form of calories for so many years.
My addiction to food. The ease with which what I ate hid my own
reflection. Maybe this all sounds like an overstatement, or a hyper-
bolized tabloid headline: *Sad, Fat Woman Juices Her Way to Happiness and a Killer Bod*. That's really not how I mean it. But when I
finally took the step to reclaim my health, and as those dastardly
detox symptoms worked their magic, I began to realize just how
much crap I needed to rid myself of—both physically and
emotionally—before I could finally get to the bottom of my toxic
relationship to food, and my warped body image.

Our bodies give us opportunities to detox every day. Even the
word "breakfast," literally "break fast," is a recognition of the fast

we (in theory) just completed overnight. When we are fasting, we are, by definition, detoxing. I began to realize that prior to this juice fast, each morning after my "overnight fasts" (a.k.a. "sleep"), as soon as I would get my morning lull or headache, I would immediately go for the coffee—because I needed caffeine to stave off the detox that was making me feel like crap. Shockingly, this is not that dissimilar from detoxing from drugs or alcohol. As soon as we feel the shakes, we need our fix, and then it is magically all better. It's why I always knew instinctively that when I got cranky, the solution would be a lovely bowl of sugary cereal. When we consume foods that don't nourish us, we are keeping the toxins in our bodies, and forcing our bodies to stop detoxing. The only way to get over the painful detox period is, frankly, to white-knuckle it.

So when I stopped consuming those foods and started juice fasting, my body had no other choice but to bring the toxins out—hence the icky symptoms I was experiencing. My hope was that, once they were gone, my body would thrive. During that first juice fast, it was this very thought that kept me going.

Of course, in reality and in retrospect, I think I probably did actually see weight loss as the primary reason behind doing it, but it was too difficult to admit that to myself at the time. I had failed at that far too many times. Instead, recognizing the many health benefits—physically and mentally—made it a lot easier to carry out than simply a "diet," like the many diets I had been on in the past, which focused solely on shedding pounds. I think that the mental shift that made juice fasting doable for me was looking at it, ironically, as a way of feeding myself, rather than a way of depriving myself.

And it's true: I was feeding myself better than I ever had in my life. Funny thing. Although I wasn't eating solid food, simply by consuming so much vegetable and fruit juice, I was flooding my body with nutrients. It would be nearly impossible for any of us to actually eat the amount of nutrients we consume during a juice fast. I preferred to look at juice fasting as abundance rather than deprivation. It was a tiny mental shift, but one that made all the difference for me.

There are other ways in which juice fasting was so much easier for me than dieting. One is the fact that it has very clear and concise parameters. Grabbing a slice of (vegan) pizza, for example, could somehow be rationalized if I were on a "diet" (I could always bend the rules enough to have that pizza by imagining I would make up for those calories—those all-important calories—with subsequent deprivation), but when I'm on a temporary juice fast, the guidelines are so clear and unbending that it's nearly impossible to rationalize my way out of it. Since rationalization is my stock in trade, this was hugely important to me.

Another thing that has always worked for me about juice fasting is that I always knew when my next juice was coming—and it was usually within two to three hours. Plus, though there is unquestionably some degree of calorie reduction on a juice diet, there are certainly enough calories that I could live my life virtually uninterrupted and unaffected, except for perhaps going a bit slower than usual (and allowing a bit more time to go from sitting to standing). So even if I had a hankering for a slice of pizza, I would simply implement the tools I had already begun to create—reading the affirmation on my fridge; reminding myself of the reasons I started; tapping into the support I was finding online and with Mariann; reading books about health; finding my own brand of meditation— and I would remember that in two to three hours, I would get another juice. That kept me going when the going got tough.

FIFTEEN

—

a healthy obsession (days 6–10)

As I continued on this journey through my first ten-day juice fast, I could not possibly have known how deeply and permanently my life would change because of it. Looking back at the daily video log I kept, which documented my challenges, thoughts, and excitement throughout the process, I am grateful to have a play-by-play detailing everything from discovering new vegetables to what it was like to trade in caffeine for carrots to how I felt stepping on the scale for the first time after the initial fast.

Admittedly, there's a degree of self-involvement that I believe is inherent to anyone who has undergone such a radical physical transformation as I have. There's a fascination with "my former self" and how that relates to the me now.

"Does she look like me?" I asked Mariann, when we recently went back and watched this first juice vlog. It's a question I ask frequently when an old video or photo of me appears. As hard as I try, I can't seem to find myself in the reflection looking back.

"What do you mean *she?*" Mariann responded. "That's *you*, honey. And you were really cute."

And yet I couldn't find me in there—in her rounder face and fuller cheeks. I've questioned if it's that I don't *want* to find me there, as if there's something I should be ashamed of. But that doesn't resonate with me. When I look back at that old video—or at the countless videos from my high school and college days—I just think of how much my heart has changed ever since my body has.

Or perhaps I've got that backward: Maybe what has actually changed is not me, but everyone else.

What I do know for sure is that during that first juice fast, I began a long journey that I'm still very much on, of cleansing my palate, expanding my mind to the idea of starting with fresh ingredients to match my fresh start, and altogether shifting my focus.

It all started with juice.

day 6

One of the best side effects of being on a juice fast is that, because you are consuming such a narrow category of foods—fruits and vegetables—you start to develop a healthy obsession regarding them. You also develop a hankering to find out about new ones, just to add a bit of variety to your life.

Take purslane. On day six, I found some at the farmers' market in Union Square and, having read about it online, I immediately had to have it. Purslane is an odd thing. It's actually considered a weed in the United States and is frequently found in the wild. When Mariann was a kid growing up on Long Island, she says, purslane was everywhere—growing out of the cracks in the sidewalks. It was a weed that was pulled up and thrown away, and yet we now know that it's extremely nutritious, and loaded with health-promoting omega-3 fatty acids—more than any other green vegetable.

When I learned this, I found it astonishing how easy it is to just cast aside something that is so good for us, something that is just waiting to help us heal—and simply call it a "weed," a nuisance. At the same time, we're feeding kids milk and cookies, setting them on the road to heart disease and diabetes. When did we forget how to feed ourselves, and instead learn to listen to the lies of the food industry?

Purslane is an extreme example of a super-healthy food that just got left off our plates, but you can easily see how the same thing applies to the overall mind-set of consuming vegetables. Though it's widely accepted that we need vegetables to get healthy, I was gradually coming to realize the full breadth of their healing properties—their ability to actually prevent and even reverse disease. The potent phytochemicals found in all vegetables and fruits are incredibly powerful, and consuming them in the way that I was doing when I juiced was, I was sure, dramatically accelerating my body's ability to heal. And yet this is information that is, like purslane, unknown, unappreciated, and regularly overlooked as unimportant.

It suddenly dawned on me that, contrary to my former experiences there, when I found the farmers' market too crowded and mildly pretentious and annoying, I now loved it, and I felt particularly virtuous and wholesome as I strolled from stand to stand, fussing over my purslane, carefully examining the beautiful, multicolored peppers, and just reveling in the glory of all that good, healthy grub. Once you really get into your fruits and veggies, farmers' markets are a feel-good experience. I found it to be intensely satisfying to roam from stand to stand, finding out what was new, seeing what was in season, and stocking up on piles of brightly colored veggies. I noticed that right across the street from my favorite apple stand was a Starbucks, and I was pleased when I noticed I had (almost) no craving for my go-to grande soy latte. The vegetables that filled up my tote bag and my afternoon plans were making me feel truly satisfied, and the folks all around me with greens spilling out of their own tote bags and passion equal to mine made me feel like part of a community. These days, I continue to look forward to my farmers' market sprees—even though they are still too crowded for my taste, and often pretty expensive, and, let's face it, frequently a bit pretentious.

That said, I most certainly do not eat locally all the time, nor do I think it's necessary to do so in order to get delicious or high-quality produce, which you can find in most supermarkets. Also, when I juice fast, I enjoy consuming nonlocal produce, too, since I am a voracious fan of goodies like pineapples, oranges, and mangoes, all of which make absolutely mouthwatering juice. So, just as with organic food, I try to include a balance of locally produced foods and some tropical delights that I wouldn't be able to get otherwise. They're all incredibly good for you, and each has its own special mix of nutrients to enhance your physical well-being. No matter where I am shopping, I love the very process of picking up fruits and vegetables, and I like to imagine all their healing properties just waiting to pour through me.

So I grabbed my purslane with glee, along with as many other vegetables as I could carry, and hurried home to make soup. Yes, *soup*. (Radical, I know.) I was far enough into my juice fast that the idea that for "dinner" I was about to make a "soup-type juice"— which Mariann and I would eat with *spoons* and not *straws*—was making me absolutely giddy. I wasn't into the idea of planning my juices far in advance, so I read a few recipes online and then decided I had enough of an idea of how to make a juice-soup to throw caution to the wind and try my very best. Even more exciting, I decided to put cilantro in there. (I adore cilantro. I know some folks are horrified by it and think it tastes like soap. That aversion to cilantro is actually genetic—you either love cilantro or you don't. I'm so sorry for those who don't. But, more for me, I suppose.)

One more note about day six: The fatigue was getting better, for both me and Mariann, who had been even more tired than I was. But we both still felt that our stamina was on the low side. Even getting up the one flight of stairs to our second-floor apartment was sometimes exhausting. So much for the vibrant energy that other juicers spoke of! Apparently, that jolt of energy just wasn't going to happen for us. But, while neither of us was up to running a marathon, we were both able to get through our days without any real problems, as long as we didn't overdo it.

day 7

In the morning, I was still dreaming of the previous night's juice-soup, which was truly, if I do say so myself, spectacular. I hadn't realized how tasty tomatoes, which formed the basis for the soup, would be for juicing. I've never really liked tomatoes, but suddenly I craved them, especially with the delicious blend of cilantro, kale, lemon, purslane, and an apple to help sweeten it up. In the back of my mind, I knew that just one week before, I would have found my juice-soup to be odd, or tasteless, or even unpleasant. I was amazed that my tastes had changed so quickly, and that I could be satisfied, even thrilled, by foods that for my whole life I would have rejected. This was one of the most important lessons of this first juice fast: *Tastes change.*

I was also still ruminating on my most recent farmers' market experience and about the fact that it really was pretty pricey. Even produce in the grocery stores, if it was any good and there was any kind of variety, was on the expensive side. This started me thinking about privilege, and, in my vlog for that day, I talked about it:

> *I'm doing a juice fast as a means of healing myself, and all the while I'm abundantly aware that there are loads and loads of people who really need to be doing this, but can't afford to. Their insurance companies don't cover things like fresh fruit and vegetables because [these companies are] too busy pumping people full of drugs and things that mask the symptoms and perpetuate the problem. So many doctors and pharmaceutical companies are ignoring the fact that the best way to overcome myriad diseases like high blood pressure and high cholesterol and certain cancers and obesity is by the diet—and by adopting a healthy, plant-based, vegan diet. Even the American Dietetic Association has come out saying that—more than once—a healthy vegan diet is the best possible way to be.*

And it's not just that a healthy diet can help you "overcome" health problems. When Mariann and I had sat down a few weeks prior and watched *Fat, Sick & Nearly Dead*, the film that started us down the juice road, I realized that even healthy people can get a great deal out of a juice fast. You don't actually have to be fat, sick, or nearly dead to reap the benefits. And yet, for so many people, produce is a huge expense—especially for the amount of produce needed to juice fast.

I found that fact incredibly frustrating, and it's clear from my vlog that I was actually becoming pretty furious: "Pharmaceutical companies are too busy spending the millions and millions of dollars on things like steroids and other drugs when they could be putting it into campaigns to raise awareness about the importance of plant-based foods," I said. "Maybe they could even subsidize some of that." To be completely honest, I'm still furious. Something about that mind-set was eerily familiar, making me recall with disdain and sadness my unfortunate experiences being wrongly medicated at the hands of doctors who did not look deeply enough at my situation, finding it easier to throw an inappropriate dose of a "mood-stabilizing" medication my way than to properly assess and care for my depression.

I am certainly not throwing these medications—or other pharmaceuticals—under the bus here. Even now, since my grandmother died, I carry around a bottle of Klonopin, which I take perhaps two times a year when my anxiety becomes extreme—and I find great solace in the fact that these little pills are there for me if and when I need them. I'm simply saying that our culture has become entirely used to the idea that "there's a pill for that," and totally divorced from the possibility that there might be a more systemic issue going on, and perhaps a more holistic means of dealing with it. Not to oversimplify, but there is absolute legitimacy in the healing power of plant foods—a loaded subject area, which only a select few doctors will touch. I guess the medical industry and the pharmaceutical industry are a bit too entangled in the sheets: too busy rolling around in the sack to enter into a productive dialogue. (I've known couples like that.)

In the video, I also expressed outrage regarding how animals raised for food are treated, and I started thinking about how my own veganism intersected with my juicing—or whether it intersected at all. My whole reason for going vegan in the first place was because I realized that animals matter, they suffer, they are capable of loving their lives, and it's completely unnecessary to consume them or their by-products. Though people come to veganism, or lean further into veganism, for a variety of reasons, I am vegan because I think that the way animals are treated is an atrocity. I embraced this way of plant-based eating and living because I see absolutely no way of ever justifying, rationalizing, exploiting, commodifying, or abusing them for our own pleasure or profit—*not ever.* For me, veganism is a moral imperative.

Juicing, on the other hand, is motivated by something completely different—the desire to reclaim my health. I am, obviously, a huge proponent of and participant in juice fasting, and I am loud and proud about my positive experiences with it. But I don't see it as any kind of moral mandate. After a lifetime of trying every single weight loss scheme, program, rumor, and radical tactic imaginable, when it came to getting my health back and losing weight, it is regular juice fasting that worked for me, and *stuck.* I am eager to tell everyone who wants to hear it (and some who don't) all about my experiences with juice fasting, on the chance that it might help others reclaim their health as well, and so I will continue to offer my own insights from my own experiences. I hope that people try out juice fasting and find the same successes that I have, and that Mariann has. I hope they ultimately reclaim their health through the power of juice.

I think this contrast between the reasons I am vegan and the reasons I juice is a hugely important distinction. They are both investments. Juicing is an investment in our personal health and I hope everyone who is struggling with health issues tries it and decides whether it helps them. Veganism, I think, is an investment in the future of our planet, and an investment in our moral code, in our karma. I hope that people go vegan (or at least go *more vegan*, to start) not just because they see the positive experiences that I and countless others have had, but because they discover the truth about what is going on behind closed doors for animals. I hope that people discover the abundance, accessibility, and deliciousness of veganism— and that they see it as a means of voting with their dollars.

day 8

Today we ran out of produce, even though we had just gone on a major food-shopping trip. It occurred to me that another privilege issue involved in juicing was the cost of a great juicer. Both our first one—that weathered Jack LaLanne—and the secondhand juicer given to us from a random Facebook acquaintance worked moderately well for inexpensive machines, but the better the juicer is, the more juice you manage to get out of your produce. In other words, you end up with very, very dry vegetable and fruit pulp, having squeezed out every last drop of moisture. The result is that, in the long run, you save money on produce by having a better juicer. (Mariann and I eventually invested in a Breville— a new one, at that.)

After running to the grocery store for the somewhat slim organic pickings there, I settled down to record my vlog. Thinking back, I realize that the vlog was an incredibly helpful tool for me. It kept me accountable, and it forced me to think about things like privilege, and vegetables and nutrients, and then to organize my thoughts in a coherent enough way to talk about them. And, most important, I was absolutely loving the amount of support I was getting from people who were cheering me on—random Facebook acquaintances and YouTube users who were searching for others doing juice fasts, as well as asking me questions and offering me (mostly) useful information. It kind of reminded me of the support that my mother used to get from her Weight Watchers meetings. There is indeed something to be said about the power of community.

The interest and enthusiasm I received through my vlog also made me think about how to figure out a way to get people that jazzed about animal rights, and it dawned on me that juice fasts were an opportune time to encourage people to look deeper, not only into the healing properties of plants, but also into the horror of animal production—from a health standpoint, but also from an ethical one. It's been my experience that a lot of folks shy away from, or get defensive about, thinking about these issues. But just as we don't want toxins that shouldn't be there clogging up our arteries—so we need to release them—we also don't want misinformation or ignorance causing us to have a toxic relationship with food. When we're juice fasting, we're already not consuming animal products, so I'd love to come up with a way to encourage people to take advantage of that mental detox by not only learning about what they are putting into their bodies, but thinking about what they're not.

day 9

This blew my mind: Now that I was nearing the end of my first juice fast and starting to think about food again, I was actually craving very healthy foods—"which I hope isn't my body bullshit-ting me; I hope it's the truth!" I felt like, once I stopped juicing, I wanted nothing more than to base my eating around whole foods, hang out at the local macrobiotic restaurant, Souen, and incor-porate more raw foods into my diet. *Who was I?*

"Maintenance" is the bugaboo of any weight loss program, and I was terrified that, even though my attitude and motivations were different from what they had been in the past, I would follow the old routine of sticking to the plan for a bit, and then sliding right back into the way I had always eaten. But those cravings for steamed vegetables really did make me feel like something might be different this time.

For the time being, I wasn't really thinking about the long term, but was instead focusing on the plan for the five days imme-diately after the juice fast, in order to slowly acclimate my body to eating again. One of the resources I was looking to for guidance was the website Reboot with Joe (rebootwithjoe.com), which is an extension of the film *Fat, Sick & Nearly Dead* and offers meal plans for coming off of a juice fast, with very "simple" and "clean" foods. I planned on still incorporating juicing into my life in addition to eating a mixture of lightly steamed and slightly cooked foods. Following any juice fast, I learned that it's important not to jump into eating heavy foods again—even if they are nutritious. If you do, you run the risk of just diving right back into old, probably negative, eating habits—not to mention putting all the weight right back on (you will inevitably gain some weight anyway, since food will be reintroduced to your colon).

The period of "refeeding" is perhaps the most important phase of any cleanse, not only physically, but also mentally. During my first juice fast, it was a challenging time when I needed to step up to the plate and implement all I'd learned about how to eat, and how not to. This might sound intimidating, but it was a more organic process (pun intended) than you might think. I found myself craving healthful, vegetable-centric dishes. This leaning in toward the wholesome has stuck with me during each and every fast since. When I come off of my juice cleanses, I always want to eat food in its most whole form—it's like magic and like clockwork all at once.

I looked at the suggestions on the website and thought about how it was going to feel to have apples or pears, raw or maybe even baked (hooray for the prospect of hot food!), for breakfast. Later in the day, maybe I would try a cucumber salad with baked sweet potato, a vegetable soup, a large green salad, or roasted Brussels sprouts. All of it sounded utterly delicious. I couldn't wait.

At the same time, I was terrified to step out of the rigid confines of juicing and give myself the freedom to pick and choose foods. I knew myself too well. While I was truly craving health-promoting foods, I knew that there was also the echo of my lifelong cravings for "the other foods" as well. I knew those cravings were "more on an emotional and social level," as I reported in my vlog, but I had been using food to satisfy my emotional needs for a very long time, and lifelong habits are the toughest ones to break.

Despite that, there was definitely some confidence lurking in the back of my brain. I had really learned some things during these life-altering ten days—things about myself and things about food and health in general—that had truly turned my head around in so many ways. I felt committed to staying healthier and more mindful about my eating. I wanted to continue to feel better, and to work really hard to not be addicted to foods. All I could do was embrace my commitment and give it a go.

It has turned out, over the years, that one of the permanent benefits of juice fasting is that it consistently results in cravings for healthy foods. Each time I juice fast, through the introduction of a vast amount of vegetables and fruit, my body seems to recalibrate, I get rid of cravings for sugary, fatty, processed foods, and instead I want to consume whole foods.

One of the things that helped me stick to that first juice fast— there is no doubt about it—was the fact that I had set a specific amount of time for it. If I say that I'm going to do it for ten days, then I will do it for ten days. But if I say I am going to do it for three, there is pretty much no chance that I will exceed that. It's a mental thing. It's very similar, I think, to deciding how long you will work out or how far you will run. If you say you will run for three miles, chances are, you will do your three miles, but you won't want to exceed that—because that's what your body and brain were expecting. Everything I read advised against setting my sights too low, since it was unlikely I would exceed my goal. Leaving it open-ended has a similar effect, because I know I will almost definitely disappoint myself somehow, by cutting out earlier than I otherwise would.

day 10

I was completely elated to finish my juice fast! I was also thrilled in anticipation of eating the next day ("I've got to tell you—*we're hungry!*"). And I won't deny it: When I got on the Wii Fit scale that day and found out I had lost eleven pounds (even though I still opted for the setting that didn't display my actual weight—only how much I'd lost), I was really, really happy. Of course, I lost that much weight largely because I had a lot to lose—someone smaller than I was at the beginning of the fast wouldn't lose that much.

But it was much more than the weight loss that was making me so happy. My main impetus for the juice fast was that I had felt addicted to so many foods that were not good for me, and I wanted to end that addiction. And, on day ten, I really felt like maybe I had made a big step in that direction.

I feel like I can now go back into real life addiction free, for the most part. There are obviously emotional connotations with food that people have to work on—I'm sure I have to work on. It's really easy when I'm having a bad day to run around the corner and get a vegan panini . . . and maybe sometimes I can. But other times I'm going to try to consume mostly whole foods.

In thinking back on what had been useful to me in sticking to the juice fast, and what might help me continue to eat well going forward, I realized that one of the most important motivating forces was my work and my life's mission. Self-care had become so much more important to me because I think of myself as an activist, and taking care of my body was a way of avoiding burn-out and a way of taking care of my own animal needs. In order to be there 100 percent for animals, I need to be there 100 percent for myself. Getting healthy and flooding my body with nutrients was, I felt, an investment in my work.

My motivation of self-care as an investment in my work had been such an important drive throughout the juice fast. That motivation also acted as a reminder of how important it is to get my head out of thinking about just myself. This included obsessing about my appearance and about what others thought of me. Embracing a healthy diet and lifestyle was, ironically, a way of focusing on others—because I simply could not be there for them at the level I wanted or needed to be if I wasn't taking care of myself, too. Given my particular work and passion, those "others" were all the animals who needed saving from misery. In an interesting twist, thinking about my own health journey in this way—focusing on the importance of working to save them—ended up being the very best thing I could do to save myself.

However I got through that very first juice fast, the fact remains that I didn't think I could do it, but then—bam!—*I did it*. Everyone has something in his or her life like this. We didn't think we could take care of a dog, drive across the country, finish college, get a master's degree, get through that life crisis with more strength than before, run that long race, create and manage that nonprofit, write that book. Those are my examples, actually. With each of them, there were at least moments when I doubted myself. And then, step by step, I succeeded. Considering a juice fast from afar—imagining the day-to-day logistics and headaches (sometimes literal ones) of not eating—sounds extremely overwhelming, so I find it easier not to think of it that way. For me, as with life, I try very hard to just take it juice by juice. I don't always remember that sentiment, by the way. I am very far from perfect, with juicing or with anything else. But I try not to let the perfect be the enemy of the good.

When I finished day ten of my first ten-day juice fast, I felt like I had indeed just finished a marathon. I was exuberant, tired, motivated, wanting to celebrate, and ready to change my life again.

SIXTEEN

letting go of the past

can hang out the second week of December. Cool?" I was chatting on the phone with my old friend Sara—the one who had once reminded me of my love of purple eye shadow. "Or, wait, no . . ." I thumbed through my calendar some more. "How about early January? January . . . eighth?"

Sara's voice was monotone. "Jazz," she said, "you can't hang out until next *year*? I just want to get a drink." (And she didn't mean kale juice.)

I am an avid and passionate planner. I literally get all tingly at the prospect of sitting down and working out dates. I find deep satisfaction in looking ahead on the calendar and writing in work obligations, social obligations, and juicing obligations. There is no way that my juice-fast regimen would have been successful had this not been a key element in my personality, because given my hectic schedule, I simply never would have found the time to juice.

But one thing that meant, of course, was seriously reassessing my social life. To accommodate my work schedule, I learned to schedule juice fasts six months ahead of time, meaning that I knew I would be unavailable to socialize during that time—assuming it was socializing that involved food and drink—as well as a few days in either direction of the fasts. That meant I was unavailable for virtually two weeks of the month one month, and one week the following. Put on top of that my speaking schedule and family obligations, and I was left with a very tiny window to see my friends. If I wasn't working, I was juice fasting, and I didn't like to make plans during my fasts, for fear of being triggered by food if my friend in front of me was eating. Some very dedicated pals would meet me for tea, or even come over for juice, but for the most part—aside from doing the fasts alongside Mariann and finding that connection together—the juice fasts were largely a solitary and self-focused period.

Because I would avoid making other plans during my juice fasts so that I could burrow in with my juice and my thoughts, quite often the rest of my month would be overloaded with plans. Given my eagerness for scheduling, it became like a game to me. But I can see how, for many people, taking that kind of huge chunk out of their social life would be tough.

There's an upside to this, too, though. The period of a juice fast, to me, is one where it makes sense to keep my head down a bit more than usual and focus on rebuilding my self-care as I jumpstart my health. My life is frequently very outwardly focused—gotta meet the next deadline, gotta write the next article, gotta record that podcast episode, gotta do life's chores immediately. Something I've struggled with quite a bit, in fact, is taking time to simply breathe. A juice fast is always a time I can do just that, and even in anticipation of it, I look forward to the upcoming me time.

It was a very clear boundary I would set, and stick to, whether it was a boundary with myself or with my friends.

Recently, I was given a postcard—which now has a permanent spot on my fridge—with a picture of a woman with a word bubble beside her that reads, *"Not today—I'm cleansing."* This is true for me in spades. Admittedly, I have found that I am sometimes a cliché of myself, and many of my friends—who were, at first, perplexed by my frequent juice fasts—have now learned to laugh with me as I schedule dinner meetings and social get-togethers around my juicing schedule. Prioritizing my life this way might seem extreme to some, but now that I've found my groove with it—and having experienced the remarkable and consistent health benefits firsthand—it's just what I do. It's as much a part of me as the tattoos on my skin. And I'd even argue that what's actually "extreme" is not my juicing or my veganism—but rather, this dangerous habit our society has adopted of *un*prioritizing our health, over and over again, because, *oh hell, you've gotta live.*

All of this said, I do think it is possible to be way more social and active than I personally tend to be during my juice fasts. I understand, for example, that there might be parents of young children, or other people with active schedules, who are intrigued by juice fasting, and I don't want to make it seem like it would be impossible to do both—it wouldn't. I have met many mothers and fathers, teachers, and those working in various service industries or who have physically taxing jobs and have to remain totally on their game in order to do their day-to-day commitments, who are juicing-curious. For those people, I would simply advise working more personal time into your daily regimen than usual, and trying as well as you can to reduce your exposure to triggers (like food) and overexertion (maybe skip your advanced yoga class

during your juice fast—opt instead for a restorative yoga session).
We each have to find our own beat and do the best we can. I love
what economist George Stigler says: "If you never miss a plane,
you're spending too much time at the airport."

Despite my planning, there were definitely times when, for whatever reason, I did have to socialize and follow through with work
obligations during my juice fasts, and—I'll admit—they were sometimes painful. If a work meeting had to take place, I would make
sure to schedule it at a location where I could get an herbal tea (which
I began to allow myself on my fasts). Still, being around food felt
triggering to me. It's not as though I would have broken the fast and
eaten the food, but minimizing the outside distractions as much as
possible—which includes emptying my cabinets of tempting foods,
not watching TV commercials or reading ad-heavy magazines, and
avoiding going to cafés as much as I could—was something that
helped me tremendously. Whenever possible, I would avoid these
situations, but there were times when that became impossible, and
during those times, I just kept that saying in my head (and sometimes
printed out, on a sheet of paper, in my pocket): *The frustration is temporary. What you are doing is so good for you—both physically and mentally.
The results will pay off. Just get through this.* I tend not to be an affirmation-
type person in general, yet keeping affirmations like that on hand
was something I found grounding.

Seem tough? How can you possibly throw your hands up in
the air and change your plans for a week and a half when there's
so much fun to be had, and—once again—*you've gotta live, right?*

Yeah, you do. And living is exactly what I am doing—also in
spades—both in terms of basking in my exciting, delicious, and
fulfilling life, while at the same time prioritizing my well-being and
health. Not to sound too crunchy, but I strongly believe that the

foods I eat directly relate to the energy I put out into the world. When I'm eating more consciously, I find that I more easily extend that intentionality to my relationships with others. Once I started taking the time to be honest with myself about where food actually comes from, I found that if I truly want to consume in a way that comports with my worldview and is in harmony with my ethical beliefs, whole, plant-based foods must become the star of the show.

Financial advisers often say that we're supposed to pay ourselves first. Even in regard to the nonprofit that I founded and run with Mariann, Our Hen House, I have learned the difficult but valuable lesson that in order to make it a sustainable enterprise, I have to be fairly paid. "But it's a labor of love!" I would tell my board of directors, who gently insisted that in order to be professional, we had to move beyond just a "basement operation," and they proved to be right. When it comes to my health, I try to take that same advice to heart: I need to prioritize sustainability and self-care, within the scope of what is realistic for me. For me, juice fasting is easy. Eating a vegan, whole-foods-centered diet is even easier. Together, they are a recipe for a long, healthy life. And that is an investment I will eagerly take to the bank.

I was literally dreaming of seitan piccata—the delectable entrée they serve at the upscale vegan eatery Candle 79, which was just a short subway ride away. I would close my eyes and have intrusive images of breaded and fried wheat gluten, delicately placed atop a small hill of buttery mashed potatoes, dotted with bold capers.

"I'm dreaming of seitan again," I told Mariann. We were in the midst of our second juice fast, after finding so much value from our first.

"Stop talking about it," she responded, irritated. "It's time to have our juice. I don't want to think about seitan right now."

People frequently ask me if all I want to do when I come off of a juice fast is binge eat. When I was in the middle of those early juice fasts, that worry ran over and over in my mind: What if I lose control when I'm done juicing? Will I just hop on the 6 train and—oops!—wind up in a comfy and shadowy booth at Candle 79? What if the seitan piccata is my gateway drug back to a life of eating my way through the city that never sleeps, and never stops serving food? In the past, such as during my self-imposed "free time" at Weight Watchers, the time when I considered myself "off" a particular diet was the time when I would binge and eat whatever I wanted, and however much of it I desired, no questions asked. In the old days, with my old mentality, coming off of a juice fast would have clearly involved "making up for lost time," with, for example, a seitan piccata (and an additional order for the road).

And yet, that never happened. It would appear that the obsessive thoughts I had been having of food while I was juice fasting were their own kind of detox. These thoughts were simply stuck in my brain and my mind's eye from the old days, and I needed to extricate them as much as my body needed to extricate the toxins that caused my physical symptoms. Just like my clogged arteries that needed flushing out, my mind would not be clutter free until I allowed these images of food to come to the surface and then be set free. I would see the images of fried this and sugary that pop into my head, say to myself, "Thank you for sharing," and then I'd move on, rather than indulging. During this mental detox (which still pops up from time to time), I found out the true meaning of "free time." I was free of the mental clutter that used to compel me to binge eat. Instead, I was full of health-promoting foods, and a strong desire to center my diet around those very foods, and I had a newfound commitment to myself and to the world to prioritize self-care.

It wasn't just during my juice fasts, and in the immediate aftermath of them, that my cravings disappeared. Perhaps more importantly, it was during the rest of the time—when I was simply living my life—that I found it relatively easy to stay off the junk food. One of the keys to this was eating in a balanced, nourishing, and plentiful way when I wasn't juicing. So as I reincorporated eating, because whole foods became my new normal—and processed foods became the occasional treat—I never had to control portions again. This is hugely important—monumental, in fact. For me, controlling portions is "dieting," and dieting is something I've failed at all my life. The minute you tell me (or I tell me) that I can't have more, I want to binge till I drop. That was off the table now. When the obsessive food imagery popped up for me, I decided to just let it be. *Thank you for sharing.* Eventually, since I wasn't giving in to it, it blew away.

About two years into my regular, monthly juice fasts, Mariann got a job as a visiting professor at Lewis & Clark Law School's Center for Animal Law Studies, which was, at the time, the only program in the world with razor-sharp focus on the growing field of animal law, her specialty and the subject in which she was asked to teach. (We became giddy when Mariann was also asked to teach an entire class there in the much less talked about specialty field of *farmed* animal law, her true passion.)

So we took our dog, Rose, and we drove—using only two-lane highways—all the way from New York City to Portland, Oregon, where we lived for six months. When we were in Portland, not only did our lives become even busier than they normally are, but Mariann was working at her office fairly regularly, and I would often join her and work from there, too. This meant that our juice fasts needed to be a little bit restructured, since there was simply no time to make the full day's juices and send them with Mariann for her long days at school.

That was about the time that we found a store that offered premade juice for fasts, available in different-length programs, which, conveniently, was located halfway between our house and Mariann's office. And so, after all this time of making our own juices each and every time, we made the decision to buy them premade. This began a new incarnation of our juice fasting.

It was, admittedly, very expensive. However, buying produce is also extremely expensive (especially if it's on the organic end—and most premade juice fast programs are all organic). But it was so convenient that we decided to make it work. We took the additional money that it required—beyond the money we had budgeted for our regular juice fasts—from our monthly grocery and restaurant budget. This did force us to get creative about our groceries, since planning for our juices took a big chunk out of the budget, but the good thing about eating vegan is that there are so many low-cost, super-healthy staples—such as grains, dried beans, nuts and seeds, and frozen fruits and vegetables.

The premade juice fasts also incorporated something we hadn't ever included before—the addition of fats. Each of the daily allotments of juice that the Portland shop's program provided concluded with a nut milk, such as cashew or almond. After hemming and hawing about whether we should replace those with another green juice, we finally decided to bite the bullet and have the nut milk. At the time, we were both exercising—I was running and Mariann was doing Pilates. Though, during juice fasts, we exercised to a very minimal degree, since stamina was still an issue, we felt as though the fat would help increase our energy levels and make the exercise easier.

When we returned to New York City after our Portland adventure, juice had apparently taken over the city. Juice bars were everywhere and juice fast programs were suddenly all the rage. Though they were still very expensive, the fact that there was so much competition also meant that the prices were kept somewhat accessible. We were busy, it was easy, and so, since we had been spoiled with the premade juice fast program in Portland, we continued buying them (as opposed to making them). We still experienced the same benefits from juicing, and our lives became easier in that we no longer had to spend all that time making juices and cleaning the juicer (which, let me tell you, is not nothing).

In retrospect, I'm glad that I started off our juicing, for the first couple of years, solely making them, not buying them. It allowed me to become intimately involved with which fruit and veggie combos work and which don't. I enjoyed the process, and I would recommend that anyone interested in juicing follow suit and make—not buy—the juices, at least at the beginning, if that's feasible. But when our juicing evolved, when our bodies evolved, and when our workload evolved—and we started to buy programs rather than making the juices ourselves—I embraced that as the next step for us.

Yet another evolution for our juicing was in store for us. About a year after returning to New York City from Portland, we began to incorporate blended smoothies into our juice fasts as well (made with a blender as opposed to a juicer). The main difference between juices and smoothies is that smoothies keep the fiber intact, whereas juices extract all the fiber. I have personally found that I have greater success with weight loss when I am consuming only juices as opposed to smoothies, but by the time I started incorporating smoothies into my diet as opposed to just juice, weight loss was no longer my primary goal. For me, the benefits of consuming smoothies were still strong—giving myself a break emotionally and physically, and having a distinct period of time when I was consuming a significant amount of vegetables and fruit. Plus, making smoothies was much easier than making juices. It was something we could quickly do ourselves, and it was more cost-effective than juicing because it required less food to make a substantial and healthful smoothie.

Although my juice regimen changed as my goals did, the basic gist of it remained the same—and, like any other relationship, we evolved together.

So why do juice fasts work? Or should I say, why do they work *for me*? Well, physically speaking, part of the reason I lost weight from them was for the simple reason that they restrict calories. Ignoring that fact would be ridiculous (and yet I feel that a lot of the marketing material about juicing does choose to ignore it). Given this caloric restriction, weight loss is kind of inevitable on a juice fast, at least if you make the juices heavy on greens and you don't add in highly caloric nut milks. (And not to state the obvious, but if you go straight back to your old, crappy eating habits after that last glass of juice, you'll certainly gain it back.)

But aside from the calorie restriction, a big part of the reason I found juice fasting to be so successful was because weight loss was just one tiny part of the benefit I reaped from it. Each juice fast I did became a way to get closer to myself, to have more time in my head to explore the reasons I had been betrayed by the food system in the first place, and to remain present in the enormous physical change I was undergoing. Plus, having the fasts mapped out on my calendar—always having the next one to look forward to—meant that it was an ongoing process, and I was (and remain) committed to that process.

It was a mix of juice fasting regularly, combined with eating a largely whole-foods-based diet during the times I wasn't juicing, that resulted in my near-one-hundred-pound weight loss—which took a total of two and a half years, with the first seventy-five pounds coming off during the first year. After the initial fast, I was down eleven pounds. The subsequent juice fasts also pushed my weight down—at first with relatively large losses (nine pounds, or seven)—and then, eventually, as I had less weight to lose, with smaller weight losses (such as five pounds).

It is also inevitable that after the juice fast is over, once you start eating again, you will naturally put on a couple of pounds due to the fact that, when you are digesting real food, some of it, including all the fiber, will always be in your colon, on its way to becoming poop. That stuff weighs something. Except for those tiny gains after each juice fast, the overall trajectory of my weight continued to go down. The times when I was eating food did not usually result in any kind of substantial weight loss; it was more a way to maintain my health and not let addictive, processed foods become my normal. The bulk of the weight loss always happened during the fasts. Most important, though, is that if I hadn't eaten consciously and healthfully during the in-between times, I would have put the weight back on. Doing these things together—juicing and eating really well—were a winning combination for me.

All of this said, I actually don't think that juice fasts necessarily work for everyone. Many people who struggle with disordered eating or a history thereof, for example, might find that they are triggered by what appears to be the rigid restriction of a juice fast. And juice fasts are not always recommended for people who struggle with health issues such as diabetes, or who have kidney disease or are undergoing chemotherapy, or perhaps other health problems as well that I am unaware of.

And many people are simply too freaked out to wrap their heads around doing a juice fast. It sounds too radical to them to exist solely on juice, even for a limited amount of time. Although I would strongly encourage people who feel that way, and who don't suffer from problems that would contraindicate it, to commit to trying it anyway (for at least three days—because doing a one-day juice fast is very hard, since you're detoxing that whole day), I also understand that juicing is not for everybody. Some people try a modified juice regimen—having juice for most of the day, then having a vegetable-centric dinner at night, while avoiding toxins and stimulants like caffeine and alcohol. I will reiterate that if you start with an amended juice fast as opposed to a full-on juice fast, it will be that much more difficult to do a full-on juice fast in the future.

For me and for Mariann, juicing was absolutely the key to sustained and easy-to-reach health, optimal weight, and the overall balance I had been seeking for so many years. And to think, all of that was able to fit into one simple mason jar. Sometimes the answers are so incredibly obvious. We just have to take the first sip.

What was crucial to both losing the weight and, afterward, maintaining my weight loss and my health wound up being a mixture of my intermittent juice fasting and following a mostly whole-foods-based eating regimen. For me, one could not have existed without the other. If I had continued to eat high-fat, processed foods in between my juice fasts, I would have inevitably put my weight back on in between each cleanse. And had I not juice fasted as part of my whole-foods-based diet, the cravings—both emotionally and physically triggered ones—would have crept back into my life, and my imbalanced eating would have eventually resumed. For me, this pairing of juicing with whole-foods-based eating was the recipe for success, balance, happiness, and optimal health.

I began to crave and eat all I wanted of the widest array of plant-based whole foods you could imagine: leafy greens like kale, collards, and mustard greens; root vegetables like sweet potatoes and carrots; beans like chickpeas, mung, black, and pinto (and bean-derived foods like tofu and tempeh); whole grains like quinoa, amaranth, millet, and oats (though, sadly, I gain weight so easily that I find it helps me to limit the grains); and small amounts of healthy fats like almonds, avocados, and nut butters.

One of my first major purchases to support this new way of eating was a Vitamix super-high-powered blender. For dessert, I would regularly blend frozen fruit—cherries are my personal favorite—and make a healthy, satisfying, one-ingredient soft serve. I tried, and soon learned to love, Mariann's go-to morning drink of unsweetened cocoa (chocolate happens to be full of antioxidants) mixed with hot water. It's delicious (no, seriously, *it is*—I don't understand why no one else likes it!), and it satisfies my longings for chocolate (some cravings you never get rid of). I became adept at ordering at restaurants. Chinese and some other Asian cuisines were particularly easy. I became a fan of steamed tofu and broccoli with brown rice.

In order to make those simple meals a bit more palatable, but no less healthy, I would add nutritional yeast, which, yes, I carried around in my purse. This terribly named vegan staple (I prefer to use its nickname, "Nooch") is actually absolutely scrumptious, and adds a cheeselike depth to any vegetable dish.

And, just like that, the pounds stayed off, and, with each juice fast, more pounds began to melt off. Perhaps the greatest miracle of all was that one of my biggest fears, of feeling as though I had to limit what I consumed—that I had to deprive myself—turned out to be bogus. My appetite had always been, to say the least, hefty, and the fact is, I'm not sure that really changed with my newfound way of eating. I have always loved to eat heaping portions, and I still do. But instead of consuming heavy, oily, processed foods, I changed my "normal" foods to vegetables, beans, and fruits—and I could suddenly eat pretty much as large a portion as I wanted without the weight coming back on. Portion control (or attempts at portion control that inevitably failed) was over.

What was more, my tastes and cravings followed suit. Much to even my own complete shock, for the first time in my life, I did not feel deprived. Sure, sometimes I wanted cupcakes and bagels, but I didn't *crave* them unendingly. I knew that having my cake and eating it, too, was indeed a possibility, and that I didn't have to wrestle with whether or not I would want a second, third, or fourth slice. I was in charge of whether I ate these foods or not. Miraculously, they didn't own me anymore.

I also started to rely less on takeout and started to cook a little. I like to think that I developed into a creative and curious cook—though I never followed complicated recipes. Most of the dishes I made were prepared on the stove, from simple ingredients that were on hand. Some of these Jasmin specialties, as Mariann will attest, were more successful than others. But none of them were actually bad. Simple food is actually pretty hard to ruin, and pretty easy to master.

I traded in sautéing in oil for easy, water-based sautés (I know this is shocking, but it actually works). I put vegetables at the center of my plate and explored health-promoting sauces and gravies that were flavorful and umami rich (in other words, savory and substantial). I loved topping simple veggie and bean dishes with various versions of the easy blended sauces in Christy Morgan's cookbook, *Blissful Bites,* which focuses largely on mixing things like miso, "Nooch," tahini, and sometimes a bit of maple syrup for sweetness.

My meals were colorful and filling and full of phytonutrients and antioxidants. If I wasn't full after eating, I had more. I found that I could eat all I wanted and not worry about packing on the pounds. In fact, by putting unprocessed, whole foods at the center of my plate—combined with my intermittent juice fasts (which evolved to include blended smoothies)—I lost weight without even thinking about it. And, all the while, my dishes were delicious and satisfying. Instead of counting calories or points, I counted the happy moans and proclamations of "delicious!" uttered by those I fed—like Mariann, who became a big fan of my (uncomplicated, instinctual) cooking.

The next time I went for a physical was the following summer, after first beginning my juice fasts. Two weeks after my appointment—on August 18, 2011—I returned for my test results. My unexcitable doctor told me to have a seat. There was a Diet Coke on his desk, which he intermittently sipped as he stared at my test results on his computer.

My triglycerides were optimal at 108, he reported, and my weight was already down by nearly seventy-five pounds. I sat motionless and quietly asked him to please repeat my triglyceride level. He did, informing me that I had a "clean bill of health." For several seconds, I didn't utter a word. Finally, my doctor looked up from his computer—for the first time since I'd walked in—and asked if I was okay. I nodded furiously, trying but failing to hide the tears that surfaced. I had obviously already known that I'd lost the weight, but what became evident to me at that moment was all that I had gained—namely, a sense of control and, literally, a new lease on life. "Yes, I am okay," I finally said, meaning it like never before.

None of this is to say that I was (or am) "perfect" in my new, healthy habits. And none of this is to say that I didn't (and don't) still enjoy a good cupcake (or vegan bologna sandwich) every now and again. But making the basis of my diet unprocessed whole foods, and eating them abundantly and unapologetically, shifted my desires permanently, and—for the first time—my eating, and my mind-set about my eating, was under control. Being vegan, eating health-fully, and juice fasting intermittently is my key to remaining thin, healthy, satisfied, and joyous. My life is by no means about deprivation—it is about abundance, pure and simple.

They say the proof is in the pudding. In my case, that pudding was made out of tofu and sweetened only moderately with dates. But just like success, balance, and good health—there was noth-ing more delicious.

Though I didn't think of it at the time, the fact that I went vegan before I ever tried to clean up my diet for real actually helped me a lot, since eliminating animal products was one extra hurdle I didn't have to jump when I started juicing and eating whole foods. My first transition—the one to veganism—was made much easier by simply replacing the foods I was used to eating with the plant-based alternatives. But while the vegan versions of traditionally animal-based foods are still healthier, and certainly much more compassionate, than their animal-based counterparts, vegan sausages (you can't beat Field Roast), vegan bologna, vegan cheese (I know what you're thinking, but vegan cheese has really come around in recent years), and vegan ice cream (there are way too many to name—but I'm a fan of So Delicious's coconut-based version) are hardly "health foods."

The transition from junk food vegan to healthy eating wasn't automatic. Just as there was a time when I would have decried the idea of leaving meat off the plate, after going vegan I was sure that leaving off the meat *replacement*—the plant-based alternative—was simply masochistic. The same held true for the oily, processed foods that made up the bulk of my every meal (fried spring rolls, heavy pastas, heaping portions of rich Indian foods, French fries, New York bagels with two inches of Tofutti cream cheese) as well as the decadent, sugary desserts that I was addicted to (several slices of Peanut Butter Bomb cake, a box of gooey fudge, a bag of chocolate chips, a row of Oreos—which, yep, are vegan).

The good news here is that there is an alternative to literally every single kind of animal product out there—including those central to the Standard American Diet—so anyone claiming that veganism is about deprivation should think again. And, I'd argue, a vegan junk food diet is still a thousand times healthier than a meat-based one—since even the most "sinful" vegan food doesn't carry nearly as great a risk of causing disease as does a junk food diet that is saturated with animal-derived foods—especially if we're talking about heart disease. Like lots of things, if vegan junk foods are consumed in moderation, and consciously—as opposed to being mindlessly shoveled down your throat as if you were in a (vegan) hot dog eating contest—they are not only harmless, but they're pretty fantastic. However, as is typical for addicts, I had taken them to an extreme, and what should have probably been my "sometimes" foods became my "every time" foods.

Thus, as I proved all too well, it is more than possible to be an unhealthy vegan. It is possible, in fact, to be an obese vegan. And it is certainly possible to be a vegan with triglyceride levels that are a cause for concern.

But vegans don't have heart disease! one may think. Au contraire. An imbalanced diet is an imbalanced diet—and even veganism didn't cure my unhealthy mind-set around food. I had simply replaced a diet heavy in processed junk foods with the vegan versions of those processed junk foods—all the while feeling virtuous, because no animals were harmed in the making of my meal.

It wasn't until I took the next step and started to flood out these "transition foods" with an abundance of cooked and raw vegetables with scrumptious sauces, whole grains (the darker, the more nutritious), beans (which are also budget friendly), and healthy fats like nuts, seeds, and avocados that I really started to get healthy.

There's another reason that going vegan first, and only later focusing on health, was the right thing for me. Going vegan proved to me, without any shadow of a doubt, that food is indeed the most personal political act there is. And personal politics begins with what (and whom) we consume. I myself needed to wake up to the horror of animal production, and refuse to look away—looking away would have been the easier thing to do. I had to see what that kind of blindness was doing to me on a foundational level—how it was making me live my own life with some degree of blindness toward my own personal issues. And though I went vegan long before I reclaimed my health, the final piece for me was transitioning my diet from junk food vegan to whole-foods-based vegan (with occasional dips into the delicious world of seitan piccata). I needed addiction out of my life, and, for me, that meant going back to basics.

But my journey wasn't over. You might argue that it was just starting. Becoming thin brought with it a whole new way of reexamining my life. Everything was upside down, once again. The world was so vastly different to me when I became thin, so that even though I had finally begun to trust myself, I started to lose my trust of virtually everybody else. As I got acclimated to a new way of eating, and as my new body changed the way the world viewed me—and the way I felt within my own skin—I found that physical toxins and pounds were not the only things I was shedding. I was also shedding preconceived notions of myself and of the world around me.

SEVENTEEN

—

a new definition

To put it mildly, sports have never been my forte. This had nothing to do with being fat.

I distinctly recall being in second grade, when I was a relatively normal-sized girl, on a day that had been designated a "field day"—which meant that students were forced to do various physical activities on the blacktop while everybody else sat in a gigantic rectangle and watched. For my class's part, each student was supposed to dribble a basketball from one side of the pavement to the other—a seemingly simple activity that I just could not figure out. Every time I pushed the ball down, it rolled away defiantly, and I ran after it frantically. And so while my seven-year-old peers successfully mastered the art of making the ball bounce back up just in time for them to push it back down— making their way to the other side of the blacktop in no time—I made it approximately five feet from the beginning of the dribbling journey, having spent the whole time running in every direction after the getaway ball that just didn't want to be anywhere near me or my wounded pride.

And thus began a lifelong trajectory of loathing gym and, thus, exercise in general.

No, exercise and I have never been friends. Chubby girls who are already disdained by their peers and terrible at sports are not generally the ones who get chosen first for the dodgeball team. Once I was old enough, I masterfully feigned cramps to my gym teachers (who just as masterfully feigned belief in my fake cramps) to get out of PE whenever I could. I had zero interest in moving my body around a ball field or a gymnasium, just so that it could jiggle and bounce while other kids pointed and laughed.

Even as a young girl, that particular brand of taunting—the kind that occurred while my body was there for all to see, and while I was being forced to do something at which I had no skill or talent—stung hard. By middle school, when the others around me in gym would hoot and guffaw as I'd fall down trying to catch a Frisbee, or be so out of breath while running that I would keel over panting and grabbing at my side, it slowly came to me that my body was not mine. It was, apparently, *theirs*, to discuss and make fun of as they pleased.

Sadly, as is the case for so many of us who grew up hating gym (and I would venture to guess there are a lot more of us than we realize), this version of hell was my first foray into the world of exercise, and it informed my opinion about both sports and my own ability level for the next three decades. "Oh, I'm terrible at sports," I'd say, even into my adulthood. Or, "Yeah, I am completely uncoordinated." These statements were definitive; it was what it was. There was no room for or interest in further exploration of the matter. *I sucked*—that was all. (Thanks for that, Education Industrial Complex!)

Around the time of our first juice fast, Mariann and I read that article about Nintendo's Wii Fit game. Approximately ten minutes later, we left the apartment to go buy one. What resonated the most for us was the idea that this so-called game was redefining exercise, and it allowed the consumer the safety (and fun?) of doing it in his or her own space, curtains tightly drawn. And, impressionable consumers that we are, we bit.

An hour after that, after hooking up the Nintendo Wii console (we had to buy that, too . . .) and popping in the Wii Fit disc, we were each immediately encouraged to create an adorable avatar that strongly resembled us. The point of the Wii Fit was that—through a series of wires and boards—we would be able to work out our little avatars by making our very own heart rates go up.

Being a child of the eighties, video games were indeed my speed. I was hoping that I would be able to use this fact as the impetus to connive myself—to convince myself that I was just playing a game, when, in fact, I was working out. According to the instruction manual, which I read front to back, the games that little cartoon Jasmin would soon play would include running through a beautiful countryside, biking on a lovely island, skiing through a winter wonderland, hula hooping, and doing balancing games and yoga poses. My avatar would see more of the world than I ever would.

There were some initial surprises, however, that absolutely floored me—forcing me to look at myself more honestly, by way of my avatar, than I had ever looked at myself when gazing at the real me. Honest moments of self-reflection can come at the strangest times, truly. I had no idea that a little cartoon version of me would make me open my eyes. Truthfully, I wasn't ready for it. My bubble of denial—my refusal to see myself as the size I actually was—ultimately popped when the Nintendo gods, who eagerly weighed me each time I stepped on the exercise platform, declared me "obese" and made my avatar go from the default, pencil-like size to a huge, round tomato size. Even though the only people in the room were me and Mariann, the glaring truth on my TV screen—the flippant and coldhearted way the computerized voice called me "obese"—shattered and humiliated me.

Here's how it happened: On that first day, I stepped on the Wii Fit scale and heard a series of beeps, as my cute avatar that I had just created—complete with my black hair in a chic do and thick-framed black glasses—spun in dramatic circles, magically propelled off the ground. Then the beeping slowed and finally stopped, and the high-pitched, computerized voice disapprovingly chirped those words, "That's obese," sending avatar-me into a rapidly expanding motion that seemed to be a surprise even to her. I stared at the screen with my mouth wide open, and she stared back at me. We were reflections of one another, and I suddenly didn't know which one was real. I did, however, know that it was time to draw the blinds and go skiing.

"Obese" was the word that the Nutrisystem employee had used when she spoke past me and to my TM all those years prior. "She's obese," that woman had said, as if I were a prized pig up for auction. And though I always knew I was plump, it wasn't until I lost the weight and looked at old pictures of myself that I realized just how large I used to be. It shocks me to no end how many untruths we are capable of convincing ourselves of. (In truth, it makes me wonder what I am not seeing about myself these days, and that thought makes me shudder.) Perhaps I should be grateful to the callous, cold Wii Fit robot voice for giving it to me straight.

During my initial juice fasts, and at the times in between, my Wii Fit kept me good company—despite my hard feelings about its initial judgment. Mariann, of course, had created an avatar version of herself, too—with brown wavy hair and big blue eyes—but her avatar was simply "overweight," and not nearly as round as avatar-me.

(On one night when we were apparently loopy from our overconsumption of kale juice, we concluded that since we had decided we would never have kids, we would create an avatar kid. An avatar child, it turns out, requires far fewer resources from the planet and is much cheaper to put through college. Mariann and I combined our best physical features—my thick black hair with Mariann's blue eyes; my freckles with Mariann's cute ears—and, voila, there was "Mavis," our darling little girl.)

My plan worked. After joining the Wii Fit bandwagon, I successfully managed to trick myself into exercising by telling myself I was just playing games. (And now I also needed to be a good role model for Mavis.) Though I'm not sure that anything I did with the Wii was especially exerting, it did manage to effectively put me into my body in a way I hadn't ever been. I found myself proud of the beads of sweat that would collect on my forehead, and I eventually even invested in a sports bra—the first I had ever owned.

I don't really attribute my weight loss to my exercising (though I'm sure it didn't hurt). No, my key to weight loss was not my fake hula hooping—but moving my body gave me a newfound "ownership" of myself that had previously been lost all those years ago while I was failing to dribble my ball across the unforgiving blacktop.

Just one year later—after losing seventy-five pounds—I shocked myself by agreeing to try out running (like, as in, actually *outside*) alongside a similarly skeptical but nonetheless motivated Mariann. It had been Mariann's idea, actually, and was partly spurred by her recognition of my frenetic energy that developed as my pounds came off. She knew I had to do something to expel this new buzzing electricity, which frequently caused my legs to unendingly bounce up and down, or me to speak quickly and tirelessly. Unlike when I had been heavier, losing weight gave me an inordinate amount of get-up-and-go. Yet I had nowhere to go *to*, because when I exercised—which was still only sporadically—it was still centered around my Wii Fit. (Notably, as I lost weight, my me-avatar got more svelte, too, which she seemed quite pleased about. I know I was.)

And so I told Mariann I would try it. Part of my own motivation—aside from the undeniable fact that I had a significant amount more energy at this lighter weight—was that I was fearful that my frequent juicing was negatively affecting my metabolism. Plus, my body—though thinner than ever—was extremely droopy. As my weight came off, my skin became somewhat loose. It was mostly around my stomach, where stubborn skin would sag like a deflated balloon, both around my waist and also in the real estate between my hips that always seemed to be hanging in the shape of a smile. There was skin on my upper arms, too, which would lightly flap when I'd exuberantly wave to someone (I have since mastered the art of saying "hello!" really loudly instead of lifting my floppy arms). These afflictions were, I would later realize, going to be permanent, but I suspected (and was ultimately correct) that the better shape I was in, the less droopy the droopiness would be.

The only sneakers I had were ratty and ancient, and the closest thing I had to "running clothes" were old sweatpants with a broken elastic around the waist and an oversized T-shirt that I had once worn while painting my bedroom deep purple (it had the stains to prove it). Thankfully, the sports bra I had bought for my fake hula hooping still fit (enough, anyway) to at least keep my breasts from bouncing all over lower Manhattan.

Mariann and I decided to start with a trial run (literally)—just around the block a couple of times. We needed to see what we were getting into before we did anything serious. Mariann decided to combine that initial jog with taking our dog out for some exercise, too, but when Rose insisted on stopping at every tree, it became clear that running as a family was not in our cards. Plus, Mariann's and my pace did not match, and so we decided to put a bit of autonomy into our exercise regimes, and—from then on—meet at home afterward for cocoa and cartoons.

And so I dove into this running thing solo (just as Mariann and Rose developed their own routine of jogging, stopping, walking; jogging, stopping, walking) and thank goodness for that autonomy. Turned out, running hurt both my body and my self-esteem—and I saw no reason to expose Mariann (or Rose) to my faltering, or to the emotional burden I realized I had been carrying when I first pounded the pavement. Running simply did not come naturally to me, and I was too embarrassed for even my life partner to watch me lose my footing so easily. Blame it on my early days of gym class, but once I transferred my exercise to outside as opposed to behind the safety of my drawn blinds, it became apparent to me that I carried a significant amount of shame inside, which was attached to those moments of physical exertion. The shame was trapped in my muscles, and in order to move past that pain—or, more accurately, *through* it—I needed to first find grounding inside myself. I needed to teach myself that running was not necessarily something I would do to get away from the world; rather, it was something I could do to feel more secure within it. I could, in fact, let the shame go.

During that first fateful solo run, I headed west toward the glistening Hudson River—which, even though it was only a few blocks from my apartment, was a place I rarely ventured. After about three minutes, I realized that I would have to hold my pants up for the rest of my run, and I made a mental note to buy exercise bottoms that fit. In my ears, the soundtrack to *A Chorus Line* kept me company, distracting me from my shortened breath and my burgeoning side stitch. When images of my classmates all those years ago popped into my head at around a half mile in—laughing at my ill-fitting pants and my awkward stride—I shook them away and focused instead on the lyrics of "One Singular Sensation" that blasted through my earbuds and my doubts.

Encouraging myself to go as slowly as I could so that I would not, in the long run, burn out (or black out), I made it a mile out and then stopped—catching my breath and gazing in awe at the river in front of me.

One thing I love about running is the feeling of freedom and anonymity that it brings me. On a normal day, I am weighed down with several bags full of papers, laptops, recording equipment, a book, and even an emergency umbrella (*you never know*). But when I run, I carry nothing except my mood and my mind, which are frequently their own kind of heavy. Still, this detachment, even briefly, from *stuff* is liberating. Pair that with the fact that when I run, I have a bandana wrapped around my head, dark sunglasses covering my eyes, and music drowning out the crowds, and I feel utterly free and unrecognizable—even to myself.

But on that day when the Hudson River stood in front of me inexplicably moving me to tears with the soft whispers of its Zen-like ripples, I wasn't yet thinking about the freedom that running would unleash in me during the coming months and years, when it would become as regular a part of my routine as my morning cocoa. As I held on to the rail, panting, forcing away more images of bullies from years past, I could never have grasped that running would soon be the key for me to find my own mental balance. I continued to grasp my waistband as *A Chorus Line* still poured into my ears, forcing the passersby into the musical of my mind's eye— they walked, ran, and biked to the tune and the beat of the songs. Their stories became embedded in mine, to the soundtrack that had been a part of my life for so many years. I was, I realized, *having fun*. I wiped the sweat off of my forehead and the trickling tears out of my eyes, and I ran a little bit farther.

The following year, my arms and life both sported a new definition that I could never have anticipated.

It was still pitch-black out as I waited on the bathroom line at Starbucks, along with the other jittery marathoners and half-marathoners—many of whom sipped black coffee and munched on a half of a banana. I had trained long and hard for this morning, which, if all went as planned, would culminate with my wearing a fake medal around my neck that said I just ran 13.1

miles—an honor that would act as the predecessor to what I would consider my true reward, the almond flour pancakes I intended to make for lunch.

It was Friday, October 30, 1992—my thirteenth birthday, and the day before my bat mitzvah. Since Halloween was going to fall on the weekend, we kids dressed up on this day instead. It all seemed so serendipitous: I get to be doted on all day as the birthday girl, and I get to dress up as a cowgirl? My teenage years were off to a marvelous start—or so I thought, as I entered my middle school that morning, my permed hair tucked into my big straw costume hat.

Despite being an unconventional kid whom the bullies loved to prey upon, I had nonetheless managed to carve out a place with a very small but kind clique of friends. As I approached my locker, I beamed, noticing that these friends had decorated it with streamers and a giant card—a sweet gesture that was not uncommon in my school when it was someone's birthday. It was still early, and the other students around me were readying themselves for homeroom. I stood in awe of what my buddies did for me that morning, feeling extra special, because—holy crap—I was a teenager now.

A teenager! I had practiced being one for so long that it hardly seemed real when it finally happened. I was so happy at that moment—eager to jump into my adolescence with the appropriate balance of lipstick and angst—that I barely registered when the stranger behind me, who disappeared into the crowd before I managed to see who he was, yelled, "Happy Birthday, Fatso," and knocked off my hat.

As I stood at the starting line listening to the national anthem, I was surprised to find myself becoming a little *verklempt*. Despite the many hurdles I'd jumped through to get to this point—losing nearly one hundred pounds, training daily to become a bona fide runner—I rarely took a minute to absorb what it was I had actually accomplished. The song finished and, all around me, on that brisk October morning in Portland, Oregon—the city Mariann and I were temporarily calling home—thousands of people hooted and roared. Slowly the runners took their places. "I can do this," I whispered to myself. "I am going to do this."

"I am going to do this," I told myself as I made the bold choice to not ignore the insult, but instead to stand on the tiptoes of my cowboy boots and try to find the person who'd taken it upon himself to ruin my moment, my morning, my mood. "Who the hell was that?" I yelled through cupped hands, loud enough for the kids passing by to slow down and blankly gaze in my direction. There was no answer.

I knelt down and picked up my hat, which was now bent. From the right, somewhere in the sea of kids, I heard it again—"Fatso! Fat-Ass!"—though this time there were hoots and hollers from the perpetrator's friends.

Everyone was dressed up, so I could hardly see anyone's face. I looked in the direction of Batman and Freddy Krueger, but they scampered away—along with Homer Simpson and Ross Perot. "Jerks," I whispered to myself as I tried to unbend my hat. I turned and faced my locker and, despite my best efforts, my eyes welled up with tears.

My eyes welled up with tears. I had started the race. I gathered myself, then gathered my resolve. I needed to pace myself.

I gathered my books, closed my locker door. My friends' decorations stared back. Happy Birthday, Jazz! *said the inside of the goblin-themed birthday card that was taped at eye level. It was signed by my group of*

girls: Patty, Kathryn, Sonia, Lindsay, Neha, and Kristin. They were
the ones who sat beside me at lunch these days. We had all silently agreed
to ignore the taunts directed my way, intended to fracture me. Perhaps it
was true that I still had just as many enemies as before, but even on my
saddest days, I could not deny that I had friends, too.

Despite still feeling shaken by what had just happened, I decided
to try again at making this a good day. I blinked a few times—a trick
I had learned that got rid of swelling tears—and I turned around,
making my way to homeroom.

I made my way to the halfway point of my race—just over six
and a half miles. The sun had come up, and the initial exuberance
of starting a race had died down. In my earbuds, *A Chorus Line*
blasted. I glanced at the scars on my palms. In the past three
months of training, I had fallen and cut my knees and hands so
many times that I began to wonder if I should buy stock in Band-
Aids.

But even with my minor injuries, I had found that I looked
forward to my morning runs with the ardor of a poet. After my
initial solo run one year prior, maintaining my resolve to keep
running was always a bit of a struggle, and I often whined and
kvetched until I was about a mile into my jog, which was usually
when I would begin to find my groove. Running grew on me. For
one thing, it was the only time I truly had to myself—time I'd
sometimes spend ruminating about those, humans and animals,
who would never know the freedom I had right at that moment,
as I leapt and zigzagged through my new path.

Beyond that, running also brought me something deeply personal: It grounded me within my new body in a way that I wasn't
sure would have been possible had I not ever laced up my

sneakers—thanks to Mariann's suggestion. Losing weight created a messy divorce from my body as I knew it—and I'm not even sure I had known it all that well before anyway. I had been completely separated from my physical self, and running—much like my tattoos—started the process of putting back together my fragmented pieces.

In homeroom, my teacher—Ms. Corey—gave me an extra-warm smile. So often, it was the calm reassurance of my teachers that got me through the day.

And it was that very calm reassurance that I grabbed on to a few minutes later when the bell rang for first period, and I once again walked past my locker on my way to class, only to find that my birthday decorations had been ripped apart and my locker vandalized.

With my hands wrapped around my books and disbelief wrapped around my heart, I stood motionless in the middle of rushing students— and at the same moment that my teacher's smile from just moments before began to fade in my mind's eye, the mysterious masked kids started up again. Not even bothering to turn around this time to figure out the source of the taunting, I focused instead on the birthday card my friends had all signed. With a red pen, somebody had crossed out their names and their birthday wishes, replacing it with the word "fat," written in bold print over and over again: FATFATFATFATFATFATFAT.

From behind, the voices jeered me.

Up ahead, my friends cheered me. Michelle, Debbie, and Beth were standing at the finish line, which was just a few feet in front of me now—and where they had been waiting for hours, Debbie and Beth with open arms, and Michelle with a celebratory pumpkin soy latte, special for today since it was, after all, October. I lifted my arms Rocky-style as I half leapt and half limped across the finish line—the final step that ensured I could now proudly display the "13.1" sticker I had foolishly bought a few days prior, immediately convinced that putting it up before the race would be a jinx.

My friends didn't let up; they acted as though I were the first person in Portland—a running town, if ever there were such a thing—to finish 13.1 miles and live to tell the tale. They were insanely proud of me, and their outlandish excitement made me cry with laughter—though it was possible that my tears were also due to the muscle spasms that had worked their way around my left hamstring.

A teenage volunteer gingerly put a blanket around me that looked like it was made of aluminum foil. She chirped, "Congratulations," like she meant it, and someone else placed my plastic medal around my neck. I sipped my pumpkin latte and then laughed some more.

I could practically smell the pancakes I'd make when I got home.

When I got home later that day, my TM held me as I cried. She whispered, "Shhhh," and promised that the next day, my bat mitzvah, would be wonderful. All my girlfriends would be there to help me celebrate as I followed the Jewish rite of passage and became a "woman."

"You're an awesome woman," my friend Beth said to me as she drove me home. "Look at all you've accomplished."

"You have so much ahead of you that you will accomplish," said my mother. "You're practically an adult."

"The great thing about being an adult," I told Mariann a few hours later, "is that you can do things like drink beer with your pancakes."

"I want pancakes for dinner," I told my mother, through my unrelenting sobs.

An unmistakable look of disapproval flashed across her face, but I pretended not to notice. "Okay," she said, though from just a little bit further away.

I ate my pancakes and I drank my beer. My friends and my partner were beside me, and even the spasm in my leg was a welcome addition to our celebration. It reminded me that I was alive. It reminded me that I could get past the finish line if I wanted to—even if I had a few extra scars to prove that I did it.

IV

what i found

––––––––––––––

EIGHTEEN

—

no, really, after you . . .

The man next to me at the mailboxes in the lobby of my building smiled at me. I secretly held my breath, convinced that I was about to get mugged. He lingered as I grabbed the eclectic mix of lamp catalogs, tax documents, and Chinese restaurant menus from inside my tin box.

It took a minute to recognize him as my downstairs neighbor, a harmless-looking guy who had never said three words to me in the five years since I'd moved in. I used to try to strike up a conversation with him, and with the other people who lived there, but to no avail. So I gave up trying, saving my energy for more important things like chewing.

Admittedly, it had seemed odd to me not to offer the common, universal courtesy of "hi," or at least a head nod. After all, my neighbors and I knew extremely intimate details of each other's lives: I could smell what they were cooking for dinner; I could hear when they were arguing on the phone; I could easily catch

accidental glimpses of them in the hallway unloading their groceries from their "granny carts," or unloading their problems onto
their partners—and, I'm sure, they knew the same things about
me. So why they never said hello when we passed in the hallways
always baffled me. (And why I eventually took their lead and
ignored them right back perhaps baffled me even more.) But I got
over it—figuring it was a New York City thing. Folks here were
too cool for hellos, too busy for small talk. You came here to be
famous, not affable.

My neighbor was still standing there. I shut and locked my
mailbox and then faced him, smiled just a tiny bit, lifted my eye-
brows. I was guarded, but I was present. *If you want to talk, talk.*

"You just . . . you look *great*," he started, shaking his head left
and right a tad maniacally. "I mean . . . I hope it's okay for me to
say that, but—gosh, do I even know your name? I'm Christian."

I let a second go by, realizing what was happening here.

"I'm Jasmin," I responded, still somewhat guarded—perhaps
more so, actually. "And thank you," I added. "That's very nice."

"It's astonishing! I mean . . . *Wow!*" Christian was the one looking down now, acting somewhat embarrassed, one hand in his jeans
pocket and the other cupping the back of his neck. He was still
shaking his head. "How much weight did you lose? Can I ask?"

I laughed nervously. My laugh was far away. I rubbed my
thumb on the lamp catalog, wondering if they had any lamp-
shades that weren't made of silk.

"Thank you," I said again, ignoring his question. "That's really
nice of you."

And, on some level, it was.

After that day, when he would see me, Christian would go out
of his way to hold the front door when I was carrying too many

bags, to comment on the weather when we were again at the mailbox, and even—every now and then—to remind me that I looked great.

My name is *thin*. And I am the queen of this prom called *life*.

There were many aspects of losing nearly one hundred pounds that I expected or anticipated (as soon as I realized that this was something that could and would happen). Though I certainly did not understand the intricacies that would be involved, I knew that I would feel much different if I ever became thin, because "fat" was such a huge part of what had shaped my personality and how I related to the world. I think I expected that I would find it easier to maneuver myself in the world—both physically and mentally—which proved to be accurate, in a lot of ways.

But what I did not expect—and what floored me, really—was how radically differently the world would treat me when I went from the taboo state of being fat to the socially acceptable opposite: thin. I knew that I was often mistreated as a fat person, for the sole reason that I *was* a fat person. I was bullied as a kid and overlooked as an adult. So it would therefore seem normal to assume that the opposite would be true—that the world would be easier on me once I was thin.

But until it happened, and until I experienced firsthand the enormity of difference in the way people behaved around me and the attention they paid to me once I lost the weight—demonstrated by men holding doors for me where before they often hurried in front of me; women complimenting my blazer where before they blazed past me—I had no idea what was about to hit me. It wasn't until I was thin that I realized just how badly I was being treated when I was fat, and just how overlooked I was by a society that arbitrarily celebrates thinness and—in ways so deeply indoctrinated into our behavior—*tut-tut*s fatness. Fat equals lazy and lacking and less than. Thin equals "no, really, after you."

Rush hour in the New York City subway can be grueling. Everyone is in a huge hurry to get to work or transition into their evening, and so they pile by the hundreds of thousands into a maze of subway cars, often squished into a space that is way too small, surrounded by the other residents of this veritable clown car.

On one particular cold wintry day when I was in my early twenties, I found myself in the unfortunate situation of boarding the subway at Grand Central Station at the very hectic eight A.M. hour—the dreaded morning commute. Thousands of people wearing wet snow boots and hooded coats rushed out of the turnstiles, making it impossible for me, headed in the opposite direction, to scan my MetroCard and enter—the oncoming foot traffic was just too relentless. The only possible way to get through was to assert my space, to just swipe the card and start barreling through.

This is standard behavior for New Yorkers, who wouldn't get anywhere if all they did was let others pass by in front of them. You can't succeed that way, let alone board a crowded train or enter a subway station at the precise moment when everyone else is leaving and there's no room for you to get through. In short, you can't get anywhere unless you push and shove your way to where you want to be.

So I gathered the gumption to take ownership of one of the several turnstiles, forcing the people on the other side to wait approximately three seconds for me to get my turn. Apparently, those three seconds were vitally important to one particular businessman, who found it completely unacceptable for a fat twenty-something to interrupt the line in order to get through.

"You fucking fat bitch," he said—not quietly—as I quickly swiped my card, causing him a very brief delay.

It took me a second to register what was happening, and when I got to the other side of the turnstile, inside the subway station now and face-to-face with this man, I stopped in my tracks. "What?" I asked him, without actually registering that I was speaking.

He stood a few inches from me now and the foot traffic split around us, like we were two rocks caught in an angry stream.

"I said," the man repeated, overemphasizing each syllable, "you're a fat, fucking *bitch*."

With that, the man sarcastically smiled and pushed his way to exit the subway terminal and entered Grand Central Station, where the bustling crowd quickly swallowed him and his words swallowed me.

A decade gained and a hundred pounds lost later, I found myself at the similarly busy Penn Station—just a few avenues away—where that same burdened and busy crowd paraded through the station all around me. I stopped in my tracks, finding an odd fascination in the world moving around me.

"Miss, can I help you find something?" said a man in a business suit who saw me standing there.

"No, thanks," I said with an embarrassed smile, feeling a little foolish (and rude) for simply stopping in the middle of such hectic foot traffic.

I continued on to the New Jersey Transit area. I was on my way to visit my beloved grandmother, whose health and thus spirits were failing her. I found my way to the ticket line and arrived at just the same moment as somebody else, so I motioned for him to go ahead of me.

"No, after you," said the man, and I thanked him and took my place in line, letting it truly sink in exactly what my place was and how it had changed.

These are very small moments. But they are two examples of moments I began to experience dozens of times a week. Once I became thin, cashiers eagerly asked me how my day was. Cabdrivers made conversation with me more readily. And, much to my surprise, friends were quicker to make plans, eager to tell me how amazing I looked. Of course, they wanted to celebrate my "accomplishments" alongside me, and admittedly, a part of me truly basked in that. I began to anticipate and even expect it.

"You look *amazing*, Jazz," my friend Kelli said after not having seen me in a number of months—not since I began my weight loss journey. I was aware of Kelli's open mouth, her wide eyes, and the obvious fact that she kept looking me up and down. "Wow, I can hardly believe it. What'd you do with the rest of you?"

"What'd you do with the rest of you?" was a question I was commonly asked, a joke that resulted in me meekly smiling and awkwardly looking down. Though I did find it flattering—after all, I had worked very hard for very long to achieve my weight loss—there was a point when the exuberance and downright shock exhibited by some in my social circle became so exaggerated that I began to wonder how I had looked to them before. I existed in a dichotomous and insatiable state between craving my friends' reaction to my new body and, admittedly, resenting it.

That dichotomy spilled over into the rest of my life, too. Being thin has its perks—there is no doubt. And even though I was beginning to recognize the vast injustice of going from a fat girl who was either ignored or bullied my entire life to a thin person who was celebrated by a society that favors bones over bulk, I would be dishonest if I didn't admit that I sometimes enjoyed my new privileges, too—and I'd perhaps be masochistic if I didn't experience these privileges as positive, despite my unrelenting inner conflict.

Here's the thing: I found it easier to be thin. I left the house in the morning unafraid that I would be called a "fucking fat bitch." My guard was down; I was simply *me*. Unlike before, I knew that I would not need to keep my head down when I walked down the street. I knew that I did not have a big target on my back, or on my fat. I knew that now, I wasn't being judged simply because of my size.

Or was I?

Was it, in fact, possible that now that I was thin, people were drawing just as many conclusions about me as they had when I was fat, but on the opposite end of the spectrum? I was, in many regards, the same person I had been before—same obsession with eyeliner and with Patti LuPone, same propensity toward obsessing about people and polka dots, same unrelenting drive to change the world for animals. So wasn't it true that I was being just as judged now that I was thin as I had been when I wasn't? Isn't it just the opposite side of the same rusty coin? My head spun.

I realize that we all draw conclusions about people at first glance—it is simply human nature. But it was truly staggering to be treated so vastly different as a thin person than as a fat one, and this massive change in how society reacted to me—even though it was now for the better—made me second-guess everything. Even though I was thin now, my psyche was still the same as it had been before—so why was I suddenly being validated? The reality that the world seemingly had decided I was now acceptable and accepted—whereas before, I wasn't—made that validation that I had long sought taste absolutely bittersweet.

Or maybe the difference I was experiencing in the way the world treated me had nothing to do with my size after all. Maybe it was simply that as a thin person, I was more confident. Maybe my perceived change in the world's view of me could more easily be attributed to the fact that, when I was fat, I was ashamed—which one might argue had nothing to do with my fatness, but simply with my self-confidence—and now that I was thin, I put out a friendlier, more approachable affect to the world. I simply thought better of myself, so the world picked up on that and naturally thought better of me. Perhaps the problem was never that the world around me was being prejudiced due to the *round* me, but rather, they were picking up on my shame and latching on to that.

That theory could explain a lot of what was going on . . . that is, if it were not complete bullshit.

And yet it has been brought up to me more than a few times by empathic individuals who find it impossible to grasp the possibility that society at large is actually meaner to large people than it is to thin people. I certainly don't need to point out the way the media perpetuate this arbitrary ideal—anyone with eyes and ears can see that's true. And I'm also not saying that my experiences of being repeatedly subjugated as a fat person and celebrated as a thin one are the same for everybody.

But, for me, there is simply no denying my repeated experiences. While it may be true that the higher our self-confidence and the better we feel about ourselves, the more enjoyment we will get out of social interactions and the more happiness we will attract, there is another cold, hard truth. And, for me, denying that truth would be perpetuating a dangerous cycle of oppression—possibly oppression that we ourselves are contributing to.

There comes a point, for some of us, when for whatever reason we are invited to the other side of the fence, and we see things from the other point of view. For me, losing nearly a hundred pounds showed me just how readily we brush people aside—or harshly, dangerously judge and treat them as "less than"—just because they are fat. Though I had suspected it before, it wasn't until I was deemed a "cool kid" (or a thin kid) that I saw this truth for everything it was.

And then, suddenly, I was on the other side of it—looking at others the way I had been looked at my entire life.

"There was a new person in my tap dance class today," I told Mariann. We were sitting at the macrobiotic restaurant Souen, sharing an extra side of steamed squash, each of us slathering on the incredibly delicious tahini dill dressing. At Mariann's urging, I had started to take an adult tap class a few months prior. It was a hobby that I had begun when I was a starry-eyed teenager, but left behind when I left Philadelphia. Mariann felt that my heavy workload was starting to swallow me—I tend toward workaholism—and, thus, at her encouragement, tap came back into my life with a vengeance that even I didn't expect.

"Uh-huh," replied Mariann when I mentioned my new classmate. Though wildly supportive of my hobby, Mariann was not always exactly eager to hear all the many arguably mundane details about it that I wanted so much to share. (In addition to workaholism, I also tend to become monomaniacal, even obsessive, about things that interest me—sometimes to the boredom of others.)

"What's she like?" Mariann asked, momentarily placating me as she divided the final slice of squash with her fork, chivalrously taking the smaller piece for herself.

"She's fat," I said, then promptly dropped my fork on the floor. It had been a simple question: *What's she like?* Yet the way I had casually responded almost made me choke on my tahini.

The waitress rushed over and handed me a new fork. (If only every time you dropped something you needed, someone was there with a brand-new shiny replacement.)

"Dope," Mariann called me, thanks to my fork incident. She seemingly did not notice my descriptor for the new young woman in my tap class—or perhaps she simply chose to ignore my poor choice of adjective.

"You can have the last piece of squash," I said quietly, not bothering to grab my new fork from beside me. I didn't want any more food. Instead, I focused solely and entirely on the bomb I had also just dropped.

I let a moment pass, eyeballing the corner of the restaurant where I had recently seen Andie MacDowell eating a salad.

Focusing back on Mariann, I finally said, "Jesus."

"What about him?" Mariann replied.

"Did you hear me a second ago?"

"That I could have the squash? Yeah, thanks. I ate it. I hope you don't want it back."

"Not that," I replied. "I said that the new person in my tap class was *fat*. I said she was fat. You asked me what she was like, and I said, 'She's fat.'"

Mariann looked at me, finally fully present in my moment—realizing that I was shaken by this conversation. "Yeah, you did say that. Odd . . ."

"Yeah—why would that be what I noticed?" I said. "Why wouldn't I have told you that she has curly blond hair, or that she does a really great cramp roll that I'm totally jealous of?"

I didn't know if I was overreacting. Maybe I had just been reporting a simple fact—*she's fat, yes, she's fat*. But as I continued to sit there—and as the check came, and as I put out some cash, and as we started walking the few blocks toward our apartment—I realized how very aware I was of the fact that this new tap dancer was, indeed, fat. Getting real with myself now, I knew that her size was something I was aware of from the moment she walked into the class, five minutes late because she was lacing up her new shoes. I was aware of it when we were going around the room practicing our double pullbacks, one frustrated dancer at a time. I was aware of it when she and I chatted after class, when we walked out of the building together, when we said our good-byes, and when she was walking away.

I did not for a moment think that I was judging her—yet the question now loomed: Why had I noticed in the first place? Why had her size stuck in my head? Why had "fat" been the very first word I used to describe her to Mariann? Why was this bothering me so tremendously?

Could it be that it was bothering me because of how acutely aware I suddenly was of having jumped the fence? Was I settling a little too comfortably into my newly regarded role, and did that mean I was now inadvertently judging others as they had judged me? Was my choice of descriptor proof positive that I was noticing a sweet woman's size before I noticed her heart?

Or maybe it wasn't that deep. Was my intense focus on her size simply a matter of recognizing a reflection of myself in her? Because even though I was almost a hundred pounds thinner now, I still felt that if I tried hard enough, I could see the world through her eyes—the young woman with the sparkling new tap shoes and the golden ringlets, whose smile reminded me of Meg Ryan's and whose unabashed kindness and forthrightness made me want to change my ways, yet again. Even in my brief interaction with this veritable stranger, who handed me a piece of cinnamon gum and complimented my thumb ring, I realized how open her heart was—and how closed mine had become.

Indeed, she made me want to be a bigger person.

When you cleanse, as your body gets rid of certain toxins, it sometimes manifests by temporarily making you sick. That is why we get headaches before our morning coffee, or why facials sometimes leave us with pimples for a few days. The toxins need to come to the surface in order to go away for good. If we feed the toxins back to it—such as the caffeine, the sugar, the meat—we will indeed suppress the immediate discomfort, but we will be making ourselves sicker in the long run.

The signs of my detoxification were much deeper than simply zits or headaches. They were more than just physical. As I lost weight, my worldview began to shift, and my outlook began to change as drastically as my physical appearance. As I got thin, I was surprised—floored, really—by just how deep that went. And as the world started to react more positively to my physical presence, a horrifying thought occurred to me: Was my newfound thinness a way of invalidating the fat person I had been my whole life?

There is this inherent conflict that exists in me regarding being thin now, and yet not wanting to be seen as successful-because-I'm-thin. Can I shun fat-phobia and yet write a book detailing my journey of losing weight? Does it make me a hypocrite to get on my soapbox about how we should be kind, tolerant, accepting and embracing of all individuals—regardless of size or species—and then get off my soapbox just in time to request my tofu please be steamed and not fried? Can a formerly fat person like me hold any weight when it comes to size acceptance?

I was always devastatingly uncomfortable when audience members at my veganism or activism workshops commented on my size. Just before I went on my first juice fast, and just as the public speaking component of my career entered full swing, such comments absolutely flattened me. Roughly a year before that first fast, a woman came up to me after one of my animal rights workshops. She was in her midfifties and slightly larger than me. "Thank you for getting up there in front of so many people," she said. "Not enough fatties like us have the courage to be seen. I admire that. Keep on going." Then she winked and walked away, leaving me standing there lingering on what she had just called me—a "fatty." Was it inappropriate to be offended?

It was not entirely uncommon for me to be approached with similar sentiments following public workshops, from women who were grateful to see anyone up on a podium who wasn't thin and perfect. Our society sends a message to fat people—or to probably anyone who doesn't conform to people's image of perfection—saying that we need to leave it up to the *skinny bitches* to be the ones out front. This is, to say the least, backward.

I began my activist career speaking up for the LGBT community and those affected by the AIDS virus—and then extended my activism to include nonhuman animals. But the bottom line has always been the same for me: that each of us should be treated with dignity and respect, and nobody should have any kind of ownership over another. My worldview therefore absolutely includes people who are "othered" because of how they look or what their size is. And so the idea that we exist in a fat-phobic society—one that I existed in as a fat person, for many years—is suffocating. There is no reason why we should ever feel the need to conform to another's view of what we should look like.

Fat-phobia and I go way back. Fat-phobia stared me in the face when I was a plump teenager with a subscription to *Seventeen* magazine—when I'd longingly caress the smooth pages, knowing that I would never have the svelte and flat body of the woman I was told I had to be, the heavily retouched image staring back from the page. Fat-phobia was part of the worldview inherited by the kids on the playground who mocked me, and by the adults in the casting room years later who would cast me off as nothing, because I did not fit into a part or a size four.

My own fat-phobia stared back at me when I looked in the mirror as a young adult, noticing only the ripples in my stomach, the hanging flesh on the sides of my upper arms, the plumpness even around my toes. I saw only those things, ignoring what only years later I began to grasp as my physical attributes: my long fingers, my strong stance, my expressive face. My mother had always called me beautiful—I was *the most beautiful*—and yet I wanted *out* of a body that really never felt as if it were mine, this vessel that I was wrongly given to enfold my spirit, this body that was so completely different from Mom's perfect one. Rather than seeing my good fortune in inhabiting a body with which I could do pretty much anything I wanted, I saw it as an unnecessary and embarrassing waste of too much space. It was always too much and never enough. I was, it seemed, *self-phobic*.

So now, as a thin person, as a person who rejected fatness, who "overcame" my body, who no longer is a fellow "fatty" standing up for what I believe in, do I lose all cred when I talk about how convoluted and dangerous fat-phobia is? Or does the fact that I have seen it both ways—as a fat person, and as a thin person in a let's-celebrate-thin-and-hate-fat society—make my point of view more, shall we say, well-rounded?

Fat-positivity is a powerful and important reaction to fat-phobia. Fat-phobia is one symptom of a systemic virus that is plaguing our society—to throw others under the bus the minute they don't fit our definition of beauty, the minute they don't assimilate. I am all for body acceptance no matter what our bodies look like, and I think that it's a travesty how fat people and queer people and people of color and *insert-marginalized-people-here* have been, over the years, expected to feel "less than" by those who wear the badge of privilege at a particular moment in time.

So, if fat-phobia is bad, why did I want to lose weight, and why am I glad I did?

Is losing weight incompatible with being a person who is outspoken about fostering compassion, equality, and body acceptance? I certainly hope not. But for me personally, trying to embrace fat-positivity was just not enough. One reason is that I was physically ill and on my way to having truly serious health problems. Another is that (in case you haven't figured this out by now) I had a truly negative and addictive relationship with my food. But the fact is that I also just didn't feel good in my body. It didn't feel like me, just as my enormous breasts didn't feel like part of me when I was sixteen. I am, to tell the truth, somewhat conflicted about this. There have been times when I've asked myself if my wanting to be thinner was some kind of a character flaw, like a fundamental rejection of my feminism, or a secret longing to join the status quo. If I lost weight, did that mean the bullies would somehow win?

I once fleetingly had a blog called *Zaftig Vegan*. *Zaftig* is Yiddish for curvy, Rubenesque, "of a woman." I enjoyed the perceived oxymoron of the name, but secretly felt uncomfortable about the whole thing. The only way I felt I could blog was to bring attention to my size—to use it as a kitschy and compelling angle. "That's Jasmin," I wanted my readers to say. "She's fat and she's cool with it . . . *how awesome and subversive is that?!*"

Yet, in retrospect, I wonder why my size even needed to be a factor. The fact that it was shows me how truly unsettled I was about my body. I was at odds with it; I was against it. I was constantly aware of it. I didn't take care of it and it rebelled by making me fatigued, achy, and sick. The cycle continued because I reacted to my body's rebellion by feeding it crap. Given my imbalanced relationship with my body and with food, it's not surprising that having a blog called *Zaftig Vegan* was something that made me wince. The name suggested that I was celebrating my size, but I wasn't. I wanted to be thinner, healthier, and more balanced.

I wanted to be rid of a lifetime of disordered, out-of-control eating habits and self-loathing.

Thin does not necessarily equal healthy, and zaftig does not necessarily equal unhealthy. I know plenty of vegans who are excellent athletes, highly energetic, and extremely healthy, regardless of their substantial size. And the truth is, I know plenty of thin people (vegan and otherwise) who struggle with their health and with their destructive eating habits.

On the other hand, obesity can lead to serious medical conditions, and those conditions are plaguing our country. More than a third of adults and more than 17 percent of kids in the United States are obese. Obesity can lead to stroke, heart disease, type 2 diabetes, and certain types of cancer—all of which can be prevented. So while it is possible to be bigger and be healthy, I am furious that our country is getting fatter and sicker because we are being fed addictive foods that are reliant on manipulating our taste buds and desires. In terms of knowing where our food comes from and what it is doing to our health—we are being kept in the dark. When the light finally switched on for me, I was both relieved and perplexed.

Change is a frightening undertaking. Even switching up what we have for dinner can bring up deep fears and insecurities. I have a friend who literally weeps every time she gets a haircut, because it will mean she will be different—and people are afraid of changing. I can understand why. There is a lot of comfort in what we know.

By causing me to both reassess what I consume and to enhance my self-awareness, juice fasting and whole-foods-based eating set off an earth-shattering and life-altering process. It left me with a new clarity that stung as much as it freed me. I finally had a new body, which was exactly what I wanted all along—from the time I was a child and was absolutely sure that there had been some mix-up and I was given the wrong one. The complications arose when it became clear that my new body was not only what I wanted—the world wanted it, too. And I'd be crazy to give in to that, so, once again, I rebelled.

NINETEEN

a very real piece of me

don't know what I look like anymore," I told Mariann, who had heard this story before. We were in a thrift shop on West Forty-sixth Street in Manhattan, and I stared at the sea of clothes in front of me that were more or less divided by size, not having any idea where to begin. Was I a small or a large? A six or a sixteen? Should I go for the oversized sweater or the tight skirt? I welled up with inexplicable tears as I brought several different sizes into the dressing room, hoping that one would fit my new body and new life—both of which were still mysteries to me.

I stripped down to my underwear and bra and, without meaning to, stopped at the image in front of me. In the mirror I saw a woman I didn't recognize. My hair was asymmetrical and bold, cut short on one side and shaved even shorter on the other, with a long piece in the middle that swept across my forehead, possibly softening the harshness of my do (depending upon who you asked). Gray was beginning to appear at my temples, forcing me to recognize that I was no longer the kid I sometimes felt I was. My collarbones delicately protruded, making a surprising statement I had never before noticed. My breasts were so much smaller than they had ever been, and I briefly recalled when I was a teenager and they were the size of two watermelons, weighing me down. My stomach was misshapen and lumpy—and, unless someday I decide I can afford surgery, it always will be (an annoying side effect of losing so much weight)—and was lined with stretch marks like little highways connecting my past with my present. My legs were sturdy and strong from my running, and my feet were firmly planted beneath me. I felt more alive than I had in a long time, and yet I winced when I noticed the tiredness around my expression, the bags beneath my still heavily eyelinered eyes.

Was I beautiful? Was I horrid? Was this me?

I took a deep breath and then refocused my attention on the colorful pictures—my tattoos—that spread across my body as if it were a canvas.

I've always loved my birthday and have never hesitated to add to the presents by buying myself a few. Call it self-care or self-obsession, but in my opinion, my birthday (and yours, too) should be a nationally recognized holiday.

On my eighteenth, I walked over to Philadelphia's bustling and quirky South Street in hopes of finding myself, or at least finding a distraction from my search for myself. There, I wound up buying myself two presents: one claimed to predict the future, but wound up predicting nothing more than a twenty-five-dollar deficit in my budget, and the other felt like an impulsive decision, but wound up paving the way for who I would eventually become.

First, I bought a half hour with Tilly, a street-side psychic whose sparkly eye shadow, musical cadence, and bright blue checkered turban lured me right in. I had been planning on popping into a convenience store for something slushy to drink, when I spotted her—or, more accurately, when she sought me out.

"Come to me, child," she said, and I resisted the urge to respond, "I'm eighteen now. I'm not a child." Instead, I stopped walking and simply stared at this thirty-something-year-old who, I realize now, was probably a graduate of my theater program and down-and-out. College freshmen are the perfect prey animals, and I was no exception—with my thirst for a Slurpee surpassed only by my thirst for attention and validation. Tilly, I was sure, would provide that.

And so I bit. I followed her back to her makeshift psychic reading space, complete with cheap lavender incense that I recognized from the candle store a few blocks away and a hard plastic "crystal ball" that sat on a table with a plastic tablecloth dotted with drawings of chickens.

"Do you have an overarching question, child?" Tilly asked, and I realized she was speaking with a tinge of a (fake) British accent that I found oddly charming.

"I would like to know who I am," I said—proving to her that she chose the perfect girl to make a few bucks on that evening.

Tilly proceeded to feed me generalities that I gobbled up without chewing. She said I felt things deeply (yes!), that I was at the beginning of a great journey (how perceptive!), that I had a unique style that would get me far in life (I *knew* I was unique!), and (here was the clincher) that I had a few relationships in my life that were (. . . she took a breath and looked me square in the eyes . . .) *troubled.* "In order to persevere, child, and to truly succeed, you have to be bold. Does that resonate with you?" she asked, and I nodded vehemently, feeling sure that Tilly could see into my soul.

The following week, at my insistence, my friend Hazel went to see Tilly, who proceeded to give her a verbatim reading, popping my bubble and dashing my dreams. Tilly, it seemed, was as fake as her accent. Nonetheless, her advice to "be bold" had already been taken to heart.

But on that evening of my eighteenth birthday, before I knew that Tilly was dishing out garbage to young, impressionable theater students, I would have bet my eyeliner that she knew it all. And so, walking back onto South Street after Tilly took hold of my future and my wallet, I skipped the convenience store altogether and decided I would make my first bold move as a new adult: I would get a tattoo.

I decided on a nickel-sized black star on my right shoulder blade. "Why a star?" asked the burly, unshaven forty-year-old tattoo artist wearing a ratty Nirvana T-shirt.

My meeting with Tilly was making me feel a new sense of courage, and so I boldly said, "Because I'm going to be one." I closed my eyes just after those words escaped my mouth, because I was sure that the tattoo artist was going to laugh at my proclamation—just a smidge, just enough to make sure that I wouldn't notice, except I would have. So I closed my eyes instead and disappeared into my world of aspiring stardom and newfound adulthood. *Let him laugh.* Eventually, I was sure, the joke would be on him—and on everyone else who had ever decided I was "less than" because I was fat or foolish.

Getting a tattoo wasn't something I'd ever seriously considered before that night, because I was sure that it would have conflicted with my acting career. But a small black tattoo was, I figured, easily coverable. In high school, one of my classmates had a tattoo, and I remember being horrified by it. I went home and said to my mother, "How could she just make a decision like that which will last the rest of her life?" But I fixated on her tattoo unendingly— shocked by its permanence, intrigued by its confidence. When I was growing up in Edison, New Jersey, the only thing I considered permanent was my desire to get the hell out.

As soon as the needle hit my skin and I felt a sensation that was very much reminiscent of a cat scratch, I knew there was no turning back. It's like that moment you go in for a kiss with your beloved and attractive friend, crossing that line for good—there are no "backsies" allowed. Same with a tattoo. Much like my tattooed high school comrade, the permanence of the ink would forever memorialize this moment in my life, and it would grow and evolve as I did.

"You're done," said the Nirvana guy.

"That's it?" I asked, deciding then and there that I would be different now.

"That's it," he responded, handing me a mirror and holding up another one so that I could see the tattoo.

There it was—a tiny black spot of proof that I belonged to myself. "Wow," was all I could muster.

A moment later, the tattooist looked me in the eyes for the first time, and I noticed with a tenderness that surprised me then that his were a deep, royal blue. He smiled at me, in a way you'd imagine a father would smile at his child on the first day of kindergarten or last day of high school, and he said, "I hope you do become a star."

Maybe the world wasn't quite as mean as I had always assumed. "Thanks," I offered, then let a beat go by. Before I left, I quickly added, "My tattoo is fabulous, but I think it's my last one. If I'm going to be an actress, I can't exactly be full of tattoos." The Nirvana guy half smiled. "Oh, you'll be back," he said.

I rolled my eyes at him—or with him. Somehow, I knew he was right.

I wouldn't see it this way for many more years and many more tattoos, but on my eighteenth birthday when I got a tiny black star tattooed on my right shoulder blade, it was way more than just a proclamation of my intended stardom. I was taking the first of a lifetime of steps to reclaiming my body as my own—marking it with what would eventually be many symbols, pictures, and words that would connect me, for the first time in my life, with my physical self.

As a teenager and young adult, when my self-hatred would become all consuming, or when I simply wanted out of my life as I knew it, I would dig my fingernails into my skin until I bled. On bad days, I would do the same with pencils, butter knives, or semisharp corners of containers. My arms perpetually felt hot and swollen, and yet seeing the marks I would make on my body left me with an inexplicable sense of peace and calmness. I couldn't control the kids making fun of me, or the world around me trying to make me thin, but I could control my own actions—and the pain that came with hurting myself was a huge relief for me. It was like slowly letting the air out of a balloon that would otherwise pop from too much pressure. Focusing on the very calculated and conscious act of scratching and hurting myself provided a way to let the emotional pain escape. The feelings I had when I was bullied, and when I felt stuck inside a body that I didn't feel was my own, were the most isolating, scary feelings I had ever experienced. Finding a physical outlet for that, in many ways, got me through my adolescence.

Looking back at this, I am, of course, brokenhearted that the only way I knew to combat bullying was to turn on myself. However, at the time, I didn't see it as turning on myself. I saw it as a way to reconnect with myself, to recognize that I was a physical being and not just a cloud of circumstance and sadness. It made me feel real.

I am not going to say that getting tattoos is the adult version of self-mutilation—I don't think it is. In fact, I think that in many ways, it's the opposite—at least for me. It's adornment, beautification, and, most importantly, it's repair. It's self-expression, self-acknowledgment, and self-respect. It brought me back to myself in a creative and profound way that was both personal and universal. That process started on the day I became an adult, the day I decided to be bold—the day that a tiny black star found its way from an impulsive idea to a tangible creation. Once it was on me, it became a part of me. And then, magically, a part of me began to heal.

The Nirvana guy was indeed right. I would most certainly be back for more.

"More" started a year later with another star tattoo—or, more specifically, a tattoo of a Chinese character that meant "star."

Years after that, after finally delving into much more elaborate body art, I was actually concerned that I had been misappropriating Chinese culture and language (an idea that Denise, my short-term girlfriend who had effectively brought me out of the closet, planted in my brain), neither of which I knew much about. So I covered that Chinese character with a rescued cow whom I had met at Farm Sanctuary. The original tiny black star was also eventually covered with a bigger, more colorful one—but the point remained the same, and I still wanted to shine. I felt I had been dulled for so long.

One of the most interesting things about tattoos, for me, is that they evolve as we do. Sometimes their meanings remain intact—a reminder of a time in our life that was so meaningful to us that we memorialized it forever. It will forever be a part of our hearts and our bodies. But sometimes, as we change, the meanings change, too.

Throughout my twenties, I continued to get mostly small tattoos—the Sanskrit word *ahimsa* (meaning "nonviolence") on my ankle. The number *267*—representing the number of chickens killed in the United States every single second—on my left wrist. A *V* (for "Vegan") on my right wrist. Later I got a lightning bug—a sign for me of the light of truth and honesty—on my left hand. And since I had now ventured into the world of hand tattoos, on my right middle and ring fingers I got the outline of a sunrise—a hopeful reminder that there's always another sunrise and another chance. I loved my tattoos, but at some point early on in getting them, I also recognized that I was beginning to look like a child had taken a Magic Marker and colored on me here and there. There was no uniformity, no grand plan.

Then, one day, early on in my relationship with Mariann—when I was about twenty-seven—she said that if I was going to do it, I should just totally go for it. If I was going to be a person who had tattoos, I needed to own that. My small, sporadic tattoos were beginning to look and feel random. That was when I decided to be bold once again and tattoo three-quarters of my right arm. I decided on a colorful and proud hen who had escaped a cage—the angry, red bars behind her. The meaning was twofold: There was, of course, the literal meaning—animal rights is my cause and my worldview. I loved the idea of wearing hope on my sleeve, quite literally. I wanted a world where animals were liberated, and my tattoo represented that.

But it also acted as a metaphor for me. I was, of course, still fat. Coming from a lifetime of being mocked and misunderstood, I had, in my own way, felt as though I had been confined for years. Like my hen escaping a cage, I wanted to savor and appreciate freedom. My tattoos each represented a small, bold step in the long process of reclaiming myself, beginning on my eighteenth birthday and continuing throughout my fat twenties and my thin thirties. With each line and color I etched onto my skin, I felt I was my own person, more and more.

Pigeons have always been heroes to me, which is why, years after I first got my three-quarter sleeve of the hen, and shortly after I lost the weight, I decided that the final addition to my sleeve tattoo would be a pigeon in flight. The Dutch had brought rock pigeons—the pigeons that we see on every urban street corner—to the colony of New Amsterdam (now, of course, New York) as "food animals," but they escaped, and now they are loathed far and wide by people who resent the fact that they eat, shit, and reproduce. My general rule when it comes to which animals are my favorites is this: The more misunderstood and maligned they are, the more I adore them.

So my pigeon tattoo was a no-brainer, and it also became a no-brainer for Mariann to get a variation of the same bird. She was sixty-two, and it was her first tattoo—proving that it's never too late to change your look, or your outlook.

"Do you know that people stare at you?"

A friend of mine recently brought this to my attention while we were out for a run in Brooklyn. I was wearing a tight black running shirt with checkered leggings that stopped midcalf. It did not occur to me that anybody was looking at me except to maybe narrowly avoid me with their bikes—Brooklyn cyclists can be vicious.

I could barely keep up with my friend, who, unlike me, had been a runner most of his life. Even though I had been running regularly for three years by this point, I felt I was still discovering the fact that I had feet, and that they could move me to different places.

"What do you mean they stare at me? Is there something coming out of my nose?" I responded, in between heavy breaths, as I forced my body to jog slowly up a large hill.

"They just . . . do," he said. "Try to notice."

And so I did.

The idea that I was being looked at by passersby both frightened and intrigued me. I was somewhat surprised to learn that I was still being looked at, and yet a part of me was also unperturbed—*of course they're looking at me.* The truth is, I loved the idea that I was being looked at. But just as vehemently as I did, I loathed it, too. I wanted the entire world to leave me alone.

It had always been that way. When I was a kid, I coined the term "New Jersey stare." The New Jersey stare was—and, honestly, remains—the blank, perplexed gaze I would get when I was walking around in the mall or at the amusement park. Kids and adults would fixate their eyes on me for a moment too long, making me feel a mix of self-conscious and famous. Since I was a chubby kid, the easy reaction by my peers was to make fun of me—that was a clear and immediate way of dealing with my unstated demand for attention. And so early on, I ingested the fact that they were staring at me because I was a fat girl. Decades later, as a newly thin adult, when people would continue to stare, it was difficult to shed that notion—that they were still looking at me because I was fat, or otherwise undesired. And so I decided, once and for all, to give them a reason to stare.

Perhaps, then, my tattoos are on some level also a way of flipping the bird to people who look at me anyway. It's similar to acting, where the dichotomy of "look at me"/"don't look at me" is a well-known phenomenon among theater people. Clearly I like attention—it does not take Freud to figure that one out. But just as I enjoy, on some level, being in the center of the action, it concurrently makes me uncomfortable when I feel too seen. My tattoos are a very real piece of me that I have decided to share with the world. That allows me to be the one in the driver's seat, since I determined, by way of my body ink, the parts of me I am okay with being in the spotlight. They make me vulnerable, but it's a self-inflicted kind of vulnerable. And, at the same time, my tattoos protect me. They are my armor and my strength.

My pigeon tattoo was probably my eighth or ninth one, depending on how you choose to define where a tattoo begins and where it ends. The idea of questioning where something begins and ends was profound to me in those early days when I was losing the weight, transitioning from a fat girl to an anonymous size that the world ignores and finally to a size that is arbitrarily and foolishly celebrated.

And so there I still stood, in the dressing room of that thrift store, staring at my near-naked body—at this current of ripples, skin, muscles, freckles, and ink that made up me. There in front of me was the stunning pigeon on my right upper arm. And there was the cow on my right leg. There, too, were the remnants of my "old self," which was actually, I realized now, still my current self— such as my ahimsa tattoo, and my star that I couldn't see but knew adorned my back. The colors and patterns that were on me were also inside of me, etched into me—this *was* me.

You might say that the tattoos saved my life. They gave me an outward focus on an inward evolution. At the end of the day, when everything else except my eyeliner was foreign to me—they allowed me to recognize myself in the mirror even after the rest of me had changed so drastically.

There are things we shed as we evolve. We shed old perceptions of how the world works, letting new ones in. We shed friends— though not all of them—and we shed dreams, sometimes allowing surprising ones to find a place within us. And we shed skin— constantly—yet somehow, tattoos remain intact.

I left the thrift store that day with four new (well, new-to-me) outfits. As I was paying at the register, I caught a glimpse, yet again, of someone staring in my direction—but this time it was Mariann, who was also getting herself a new-used sweater. We locked eyes and she smiled, her big blue eyes sparkling like the heart made out of sequins on the T-shirt I was buying. But unlike the T-shirt, there was nothing manufactured or gaudy about Mariann's affirming expression. It was peaceful and genuine. I realized then that unlike my new body and my new outlook, Mariann's unwavering presence was not reflecting to me the things I had shed, but quite the opposite: Her consistent support was proving to me that, much like tattoos, there are other constants in our lives that we don't shed—they are as permanent as ink.

It seemed I had finally found something that was just the right size.

TWENTY

—

the best she knew how

As I lost weight, one person who paid a significant amount of attention to my body was my TM, my darling mother, who was over the moon—*truly ecstatic*—to finally have a thin daughter. I was now the real-life manifestation of the dolls she'd played with as a kid, the ones to which she assigned the role of the perfect daughter. (Though I'd surmise that her dollies weren't covered in tattoos, nor were they of the homosexual persuasion.) I felt, perhaps unfairly, that thinness was, for my TM, the final puzzle piece in me becoming exactly (or, let's be honest, *sort of*) the kid she had always wanted.

Not that I wasn't close to that before—I was darn close. And my TM had always loved me—unconditionally and frenziedly. There was certainly more to Mom's excitement about her now-thin daughter than just her own vanity. On the contrary, Mom clearly wanted what was best for me and found genuine happiness in the fact that I would be facing less adversity now, that I might finally stand a chance at being accepted. She naturally found comfort in my drastically improved health, and she noticed with pride that I was finally becoming comfortable in my skin.

Still, I felt that my TM's reaction to the concluding chapter in "Adventures in Fat Land"—my journey from fat to thin—was, shall we say, over the top. Maybe I wasn't fully giving her the benefit of the doubt, and was being too influenced by a lifetime of trying to squeeze myself into her skinny shadow, but even though some of Mom's kvelling came from true-blue happiness for me, I experienced her overall response as suspect. It was perhaps equivalent to what the appropriate parental reaction would be to one's child receiving a PhD from Harvard.

Even in public—like in the produce department at the grocery store—I would turn and notice her holding a head of kale and just staring at me, grinning ear to ear: a proud mama. Under normal circumstances, this would have been a tender moment, but feeling as though the impetus was that I had magically become the TD—"Thin Daughter"—I couldn't help but feel a little resentful. And in department stores, she would feel free to yell out across the Juniors section (where, as a thirty-something, I could finally shop), "What are you now, Jazz? A size six? A four?" I felt I was her trophy.

The day my mother told me that she thought I was thinner than her, I wanted to put my hands over my ears and scream, "*Lalalala-lalala!*" There was so very much packed into that little comment. I felt as though the previous thirty-plus years of my life had been this very odd game that I didn't even know we were playing, and which—until that moment—she had clearly been winning.

At the time she said that, we were standing in her bedroom and she was presenting me with an offering—four bags of clothes she no longer wanted, some because they were too small. I desperately needed clothes. Losing nearly one hundred pounds in a two-year span meant changing up my wardrobe repeatedly. (This was another reason why thrift stores came in handy.) And though I ultimately took my TM's barely used clothes—and was actually extremely grateful for them—a tiny part of me couldn't help but feel as though accepting them meant I was giving her permission to obsess about my new size, *the size of a perfect daughter.*

By taking her clothes and her compliments, I wondered if I was somehow validating her satisfaction of having everything she had ever wanted for me—or, more likely, for herself—by way of my smaller waistline. Finally I was thin, and though she'd loved me before, and thought I was beautiful before, her lifelong struggle with my weight had come to an end. If I took her clothes—which I did, because I needed them, and my mother certainly has an excellent feel for fashion—was I letting her off the hook? Was I somehow implying that the bullshit she'd put me through as a kid, when she shuffled me from weight loss program to weight loss program, and unendingly obsessed about her own much-thinner body in my presence, was somehow acceptable?

Though I'm sure a part of my mother felt the earth shift beneath her when she proclaimed that I was thinner than her, she nonetheless beamed when I succumbed to the clothes, when I tried on her jeans and indeed looked smashing in them. And even though the fact that my TM had, until that point, always been thinner than me (which had constantly been a defining part of our relationship, at least for me), having a svelte daughter was like finding an unexpected Hanukkah present behind the couch, in March. *She loved it.* My mother had always thought I was the best, and even had always thought I was pretty (maybe even the prettiest). But when I got thin, I truly became a princess, and that made Mom royalty.

Mom was so proud of me. When I lost the weight, she carried a similar expression to the one she bore when my niece, her only grandchild, was born. My brother and sister-in-law may have provided her with a baby to love, but I provided her with a new and improved daughter, a success story. *This is the stuff life is made of,* her welled-up eyes seemed to say.

(*This is the stuff therapy is made of,* my eyes silently replied.)

Even though I knew that all the hullabaloo was rooted in her firm love for me, it was just a bit too much. I was *thin.* It wasn't as though I had been selected as the very first vegan lesbian to tap-dance on the moon. I was not making history; I was making juices.

"Jazz," my mother said seemingly out of nowhere, as we sat together in her kitchen, letting Grandma rest in her room for a bit, "you just are so beautiful. So beautiful." She was shaking her head left and right, lips pressed tightly together, as if she had just tasted a rare and rich red wine.

"Thanks," I responded, monotone, as uncomfortable as always to hear my mother's cacophony of compliments and fighting the urge to rebel and purposefully start to look ugly just to counter her accolades. Even now, in my midthirties, my first inclination with my TM was to rebel against everything she said. When I was with her, a part of me always regressed to being a hormonal teenager. I even sat more slumped over, staring at the table with an inexplicable pout.

"I mean it, Jazz," she continued, her cadence more musical than usual, as I frantically stirred soy milk into my tea. My mother's hair was a trendy purplish-red with heavy bangs that landed at the top of her thick-framed glasses. (I joked to her that she should start to hang out at some of the lesbian bars I frequented.)

"I said *thanks*," I whined—still apparently fifteen years old.

My snotty tone did not register with my TM, who made up for her inability to pick up on nuance with her keen ability to always look absolutely fantastic and put together—even now, when we were in for the night. Her blue, high-heeled boots clicked under the kitchen table, and I momentarily worried that my bare feet might accidentally be crushed beneath them. I curled my toes under, just in case.

Of course, Mom had always told me I was gorgeous. "You have such pretty lips," she'd say, when I was growing up. "You have such silken hair." "Your eyes are so mysterious." "Your toes are so cute." "You're so beautiful, Jazz," she'd tell me, like a doting mother should—like I would, if I were a mother.

(One reason I will never have children: the possibility that my daughter or son would grow up and write a memoir criticizing my parenting, airing my dirty laundry for all to see. It's got to be somewhat mortifying and infuriating, especially when parents are just people, too, and most of us try our best. My mother certainly did, and she got quite a lot right along the way.)

Now that I was thin though, the volume was turned up—way up. Mom would stare at me and shake her head repeatedly. She continued to ask me my shirt size whenever I saw her, and compare it to her own.

"Are you a small now, Jazz?" she'd ask. "I'm a medium now. I really have to lose some weight. Well, at least our feet are still the same size. Though I guess mine are a little bit smaller than yours."

"Mom, please stop." I had zero tolerance for conversations with my TM about weight loss. It was simply a topic I felt was out-of-bounds, and I told her that again and again. Every time she brought it up anyway, despite my boundary setting, I was once again a young teenager in Jenny Craig, being fed herbal fen-phen with a side of low self-esteem. I was struggling through Weight Watchers, counting points as vehemently as I counted disappointments. I was overhearing conversations where she was calling me "matronly." I was discouraged from shopping in plus-size stores.

Not that I can actually really blame her for any of this anymore. Though at the time it was easy to point fingers, the truth is, she was trying her very best. Throughout my childhood and young adulthood, Mom had seen me in near-constant emotional turmoil, devastated by my size and my bullies. Though nowadays parents have much more support than they had then to deal with their bullied or "different" kids, I honestly think Mom was doing the best she knew how—which was to help me fix myself, as opposed to helping me find the teenage equivalent of inner peace. And her own preoccupation with losing weight, even though she was always svelte and stunning, colored my existence—just as most of our mothers' relationships to their bodies inch their way into our psyches and our belief systems. I honestly grew to not blame her for trying her best—but it still was raw territory for me, and I was uninterested in discussing weight with my weight-obsessed mom.

The way I experienced it, my mother's effusiveness grew as I shrank, and that perturbed me. "I need some new pictures of you for the wall, Jazz, and for my art room at school. The others are . . . well, you're really different in them."

As I sat at her kitchen table and finally looked up at my mother, noticing beneath her perfectly applied makeup and her ornate jewelry a hint of vulnerability, of pain—and of a deep longing for perfection that I understood all too well—I realized she was right about one thing: I was most certainly different now.

On some level, we are each just a product of our upbringing—of the people, places, and things that shaped us early on. These days, when I am frightened, the fear sits in the exact same place in my gut as it did when my pediatrician forced my legs open all those years ago. When I feel safe, I can viscerally recall my grandmother's soft and strong arms, with her delicate hands that held me until the day she died. I can hear her saying, "Shhh, bubela . . ." even still. When I feel insatiable longing—as I often do—I am ten again, sitting next to my extremely self-focused father in the front seat of his car, just after he picked me up for our weekend visit, driving down Anna Lane together, away from my mother and my room and my life, wanting desperately to merge the two worlds, knowing I can't. When I am confident, I am fifteen and am playing Mama Rose in *Gypsy* at Middlesex County College, belting out "Rose's Turn" to a riveted audience and standing in a laser-sharp spotlight. When I am self-conscious, I am in tenth grade, walking to the front of the room to get the bathroom key, exposed to the bullies and to my very own heartache. When I am ballsy, I am eighteen, talking my way into Patti LuPone's dressing room.

And even these days, when it all becomes too much and I have no idea who I am in this new body, I am a kid reluctantly getting weighed in at Weight Watchers. In those moments when I feel like a pariah who is still on the outside looking in—even though those around me are motioning for me to join them—I am a kid walking past the welcoming plus-size shop to the Cinnabon, the place

I feel secure. In those moments of confusion and pain about the way the world has changed—or, no, the way I have changed—I am still that kid. And in those moments, I am admittedly and notably not alone. Instead, my TM is right there beside me, gently but vehemently encouraging me to step on the scale.

At some point, as we get older, we stop letting our childhoods define us. (Hopefully, anyway.) As I got older and my feet became more firmly planted beneath me, I started to see my beautiful mother as more than just a person who existed in a bubble. I saw her as more than the source of my frustration. She became real— an adult manifestation of her own version of a pained girl. She was not just the woman who was uncomfortable with me shopping at the plus-size store; she was also the one who came to every last performance I was in, absolutely certain that I was the most talented one. She was not just inadvertently making very sure that I was inheriting her disordered eating and body image issues, she was also making sure to teach me kindness and empathy, two qualities that ultimately helped to lead me to a meaningful career and worldview. She taught me about generosity and devotion.

Indeed, despite everything, my mother has been a constant for me. A constant headache, yes, but also a constant rock. Our relationship has been fraught with emotion and complexity, and yet there was never a time when she and I were not speaking; there was never a time when I didn't feel connected to her on a powerful, and ultimately comforting, level. For better or for worse, there was never a time when my mother was not my very good friend. The truth was, throughout my life, her own issues about food and body image transferred to me as effortlessly as an iron-on patch— covering up tattered pieces of my own psyche that probably would have done better had they been left frayed and torn.

But, then, that's a mother's role, I guess—to do her best to mend you, even during those times when you're so broken and shattered that there's no real hope of a quick fix. My mother was not without her flaws, but I saw eventually that her own issues surrounding eating and weight stemmed from the parts of her that, throughout the years, had also been damaged and torn by our society's messed-up relationship with food. That thought has softened me— and it strengthened our relationship, making us closer.

It seemed it was time I expanded my view of my mother.

My cell phone rang for the third time in a row, so before even looking at my phone I knew it was Mom. She had a tendency to call me repeatedly when she really, really wanted to reach me. (Both she and I have always been very into instant gratification. It is taking a lifetime of unlearning to teach myself patience.)

As soon as I picked up, before even saying hello, she started, "Jazz, hi. I've been trying to reach you."

"Is everything okay?" I responded.

"Yes, yes. Yes. I just wanted to tell you—I'm so excited—that I went to my first animal rights protest!"

"That's fantastic, Mom." And I meant it (even though I already knew about the protest, because she had posted about it earlier that day on Facebook—which, yes, she was on now).

Ten years prior, a few months after I became vegan, my mother had told me that she'd "never give up chicken," largely because skinless white meat was the quintessential recommended diet food. She had been absolutely adamant. But at my persistence—and after I showed her and Grandma a documentary about factory farming— Mom agreed to try it for a month. She never went back.

And now, at sixty-four years old, she was dipping her toe into the world of activism.

"It was at the local slaughterhouse," she told me. "I held a sign that said 'Do Not Torture the Innocent.' Each time even the tip of our toes inched onto the grass, the security guard screamed at us. It was surreal."

"I'm really proud of you, Mom," I said, marveling at how my mother was truly coming into her own. She was, I realized for the first time, radiant—both in her attitude and deeper, in her core (she had always been radiant in her beauty). And so, at thirty-four years old, I found myself softening to her.

My mother and I said good-bye. When I got off the phone, I promised myself to stop acting like an adolescent every single moment I was with her, or even on the phone with her, and to try harder to be more accepting of her idiosyncrasies. It's amazing how difficult that is to accomplish when it's your own parent in question.

These days, when Mom flirts with bringing up anything related to body image or dieting (usually her own dieting—since her battle with her own body image forges on), I calmly ask her to please change the subject. Perhaps it's not the ideal solution, but it allows us to maintain a genuine relationship, and I simply cannot be her confidante around these issues. I have found that boycotting certain discussions with people who trigger me—such as talking about weight loss with Mom—does not mean I am avoiding something I need to confront. Sometimes, as with her, those kinds of boundaries can be self-preserving.

Perhaps my softening was also partly because that was also the year that my grandmother died, leaving my mother and me floundering and frantic, faced with the ground-altering reality that we couldn't possibly fill the void my grandmother had left. She was the peacemaker between Mom and me—the one we called during our daily fights when I was a teenager, who always left us feeling validated, yet who somehow concurrently managed to calmly convey the other side of the story in a way we would hear. She was the one who listened the best—to my mother's stories about her art students, to my own stories about the plight of animals, and to everything in between.

My grandmother herself changed, too, on that day when I showed her and my mother the documentary about factory farming. She had long considered herself an advocate of women's rights from well before it was fashionable, and she took great pride at being the first female in her family—her parents were immigrants and she grew up poor—to go to college (when she was just sixteen), and then go on for her master's. So when Grandma connected the dots and learned that animals were being treated with brutal unfairness, that this was indeed a social justice issue that mattered, her ears perked up and she started to bring up animal rights issues in her social circles, during games of mahjong or bridge.

On one particularly sunny afternoon, I was lucky enough to be there to watch it happen.

"Listen, Florence," Grandma said as I sat in the chair in the corner with my laptop, puttering on Facebook. I had been visiting her for the weekend and told her I'd help out with her get-together by serving celery soda to her friends (some habits never die) and making sure the red and white mint bowl was full to capacity at all times. Other than that, I promised to make myself invisible.

Grandma continued to address her pal. "You might want to reconsider ordering the omelet at the diner later. Did you know that male chicks born into the egg industry are killed at birth? Just like *that*?" I looked up at her, the corner of my mouth proudly inching up just slightly. "The boy birds are often killed through suffocation," she continued. "The birds are *suffocated*, Florence! *Suffocated!*" she reiterated, multitasking as she bid two clubs. "It's a travesty! Oy . . ."

Florence stared briefly and blankly in Grandma's direction, then eyeballed Grandma's tattooed granddaughter—me—sitting in the corner. "Honey," Florence said to me, ignoring the cards she had just been dealt, "can you be a doll and get me a glass of water?"

When she wasn't endearingly proselytizing to her friends, Grandma would busy herself scouring the New Jersey papers for any articles about animal rights, always making sure to cut them out for me. "Jazz," she said, hurrying to an envelope she had placed on the kitchen table, as soon as I woke up from my slumber during that same weekend visit, "The *Star Ledger* had a vegan cupcake recipe today, and the *Asbury Park Press* has a dog adoption event on Sunday. I thought you'd want to know."

(Frequently, those envelopes with clippings about animal rights stories also had one or two articles about Patti LuPone or Bette Midler interspersed—Grandma knew me so well.)

When she was eighty-six years old—three years before a benign but aggressive brain tumor finally claimed her life and, with it, a large part of my sense of safety in the world—Grandma stopped eating meat. Her decision had been looming for a few years, during which time she drastically lessened the amount of animal products she consumed, but what finally did it with her was a letter that Mariann had published in the *New York Times*.

The letter was a response to a thoughtful article by journalist Charles Siebert, in which he ruminated about the impact on children of witnessing animal cruelty.

Mariann's letter compared that impact to the toll it must take on each of us to be in denial three times a day regarding what—or should I say *whom*—we choose to eat, and how that refusal to accept what we know to be true affects us as a culture. After reading Mariann's letter, Grandma went from consuming very little meat to consuming none at all, and eventually she became more or less a vegan—except for a few candies that remained stocked in her cabinets. And at eighty-eight years old, she even wrote an article for the website of the nonprofit Mariann and I had founded together, Our Hen House, entitled "Never Too Late to Change the World," providing me with the inspiration I needed—and continue to draw from—to remind myself that even old broads can change themselves and their perceptions. When it comes to any kind of change, there really is no such thing as too late.

This is one of my favorite passages from Grandma's article:

That letter was, I see now, my last straw, the final step in making a decision regarding the path I must take. I declared myself a vegetarian, putting an important label on a behavior I realized I had already adopted. I now knew, without any doubt, why I could no longer eat meat. It was a declaration for my future, and for the future of the planet. Meat made me sick. At long last, there was simply no way I could continue to support the cruelty of animal production. The world evolves, and so do we.

Just before she died, my grandmother, in a gravelly voice that was barely audible, told me that I had never looked better. Her eyes were hardly open, and yet they seemed to peer so deeply into me. She always knew how to see me, even at those times when I couldn't see myself. I held her hand, failed at choking back tears, and told her that I loved her. She tried to talk again, but couldn't—she was too weak. Instead, she squeezed my hand four very deliberate times. "I. Love. You. Too," the squeezes said.

"I heard that, Grandma." I beamed. And she smiled, too, despite the weakness that was taking over her body limb by limb, organ by organ, minute by minute. It was truly a magnificent moment, one of the last we would share in this mortal life.

Ten days after I turned thirty-four my grandmother died. For months prior to her death, I would sit in my tiny Soho apartment starting at the large oak tree just outside the window, weeping, wondering how on earth that tree would continue to exist without my grandmother in the world. How would it be possible that life would go on? How would it be possible for me to go on? Grandma had always been the one person who got me. When she died, so did my biggest supporter and cheerleader. When she died, I lost my soul mate. I lost everything about the world that ever made any sense.

As a kid, when I couldn't sleep, I would close my eyes and imagine my grandmother floating on clouds with me, sliding down rainbows with me. When the whole world made me feel like an outcast, my grandmother made me feel like I belonged. As the people around me started seeing me differently, looking me up and down with their mouths agape, Grandma's gaze never left my eyes. She thought I looked good only when she knew I felt whole. She made me believe in my own beauty, but that went far, far beyond outer appearances. She saw *me*—not my pants size.

Grandma did not leave this earth without a fight. She truly did not want to die, and when she finally did, her rebellion inspired me to tattoo my right arm with the line from Dylan Thomas's poem "Do Not Go Gently"—the line being "Rage, rage against the dying of the light." Wrapped around those words is a stunning butterfly with green and purple hues—Grandma's colors. There is a starling there, too—an animal who is so inherently beautiful, yet considered such a nuisance by society, nothing more than a pest to be managed, nothing more than yet another individual to exterminate because she doesn't fit in properly.

When everyone else saw me as a pest, Grandma saw me as beautiful. And although she was indeed also kvelling when I lost the weight, Grandma's concern wasn't so much with my physical self; her pride was more related to the person I was becoming as I strengthened my voice and my resolve.

Grandma's love taught me how to fly. And when she left— grasping tight until the very last possible second, and trying to hold on even then—a huge chunk of my intuition, myself, and my understanding of the world fell eerily silent. Although there was a new dark place inside of me, in some ways it was for the better—Grandma was inside me now, a part of me that made me want to be exceptional.

TWENTY-ONE

my whole fat life

The past few years have been filled with such earth-shattering realizations and changes that I have a hard time realizing that this is my life.

I am thirty-six years old. I have been vegan for twelve glorious years, and it's been four years since I shed the last of my extra weight. Juice fasting is a regular part of my and Mariann's life, and the rest of the time, we try our best to consume a diet rich in whole foods. We remain vegan for the animals, but are always eager to discuss with others the health benefits we experienced once we ditched processed junk foods—not to mention meat, milk, and eggs.

Despite these huge shifts, a lot remains the same as before. As always, nothing makes me more excited than food—talking about it, cooking it, and most importantly, eating it. My culinary life remains abundant and rich, and even despite my intermittent juice fasting and my commitment to consuming a mostly whole-foods, vegetable-centered diet, I enjoy diverse and decadent meals—and am by no means deprived. My life, in all its manifestations—including food—is full of abundance.

It seems odd, these days, to meet people who have no idea that I was once a bullied, fat kid, and—just a few years ago—an obese adult. It feels very much like meeting someone at a party before I take my jacket off. We shake hands, make small talk, maybe share a friendly observation about how absurdly cold it's been lately, how we're so sick of winter. I remove my jacket, and: "Wow! I can't believe all your tattoos! That's a . . . surprise!" And suddenly, I'm that tattooed chick, and, with it, every preconceived notion that my new acquaintance has about people who have a lot of tattoos. My tattoos define me, at least in that moment—just as my fatness always had.

But now, of course, I could opt to keep my jacket on. I could keep the small talk small. And I could let them walk away without ever having the chance to superimpose their stereotypes of tattooed chicks onto me.

Meeting people as a thin person is like never absolutely needing to take off my jacket and show them the real me; they never even need to know I was once "Fatso." Back then, my body spoke for me before I was even able to—before everyone I met had an opportunity to peg me, figure me out, think they knew who I was and, for some, dismiss me, before I said a word. Now, I can choose when to leave my jacket zipped up, and when to leave my heart zipped up with it.

Yet the question lingers: How will I be able to see others' true colors if I don't show them mine?

One thing I've noticed is that I have fewer friends than I used to. Perhaps that's because my life has become busy—or maybe that's just my excuse. Mariann suspects it might also be a common side effect of being in my thirties as opposed to my hypersocial twenties, but who knows? Seeing the world's reaction to me shift so radically, so quickly, and so uniformly has left me skeptical. It's not as though I am untrusting, but it takes me longer to get there than it used to. I realize that it might sound contradictory to say that, these days, even though the world treats me better than before, I have fewer friends. It's not as though I don't make new ones now, but I certainly don't dive in headfirst anymore.

One important thing that has shifted is that the guilt, the fear, and the despair about my relationship with food—feelings that dictated and defined my life for so many years—are so much better now. I wish I could say that these feelings are gone entirely, but they're not.

There are still some mornings when I wake up and, before even opening my eyes, move my hand down to my lumpy stomach—to my stubborn, loose skin—pinching and grabbing at it, willing it away. These moments are rare, and they always pass quickly—whereas before I used to get stuck in them like they were Super-Glued to my spirit. And though they are also infrequent, there are moments and days of feeling imbalanced with my food—as if I am completely unconscious about it, latching onto it as if it were my lifeline. There have been times—albeit rarely—when a half of a bagel turned into a whole one, and then a chocolate bar, and then a plate of fries . . .

My reaching for that still-familiar comfort is, I guess, not that surprising. It's driven by that same manic need to look up an old friend or lover on Facebook—these people are out of our lives for a reason, but having them just a click away is just too tempting sometimes. The kitchen cabinet is only a room away.

Maybe these moments of self-doubt and weakness will never

disappear entirely. Maybe they will always lurk just beneath my confidence. Maybe they will emerge for me at that very instant when I'm questioning the authenticity of the stranger holding the door open for me, the moments when I don't trust.

But, most notably, these moments, while they may occur, no longer rule my life—and neither does food.

No, food does not rule my life—but it does indeed color it. Food does not dictate my plans anymore, but as a vegan, it does inform my identity. It brings me closer to a community of do-gooders whose arms and hearts are open to me, to my cause, to my life's mission— their cause and mission, too—and I feel safe with these folks. The discussions I have with my comrades—the strategy sessions, the reminiscing, the scheming, the despairing, the hoping—occur in nooks and crannies around New York City and in corners through-out the globe, and they're almost always accompanied by food. As with so many other communities and subcultures, food brings us together, and the accessibility and deliciousness of vegan grub is— as Mariann likes to say—the single most effective way to change the world for animals.

The difference is that in the old days, it was I who was ruled by food, not the other way around. A subtle shift, but a life-altering one, and perhaps a life-saving one. In other words (unlike how I feel about my extensive stuffed animal collection), I no longer assign too much importance to my meals. They are no longer the broken record of my brain—the ongoing loop of fries, froyo, and cheese crackers. While I still look forward to my occasional seitan piccata, and the accompanying peaceful ambience that Candle 79 provides, as my reservation nears, my anticipation is healthy.

I get to eat a delectable dinner, one of the best around. The seitan piccata, however, will not get to eat me. I won't allow that. I'm in charge of my food, and because of that, the food I choose to eat charges me, gives me strength, gives me *me*.

Thinking of positivity as a strategy as opposed to as a *given* allows me to readily tap into it when I'm becoming too jaded for my own good (which, admittedly, is a daily occurrence). Remaining positive and hopeful, and encouraging the skeptic in me to take a hike, reminds me that I don't have to be a naturally sunny person in order to see the bright side. I need to cultivate it, just as I do with my garden (which is probably a terrible analogy because I can basically look at a plant and it will start wilting, but you catch my drift). When I get too far down, too angry at the world, I challenge myself to remember the possibility and the goodness that's everywhere—in people, in nature, in animals.

I think of my grandma, and I hear her beautiful voice with her perfect pitch belting out, "You've got to accentuate the positive, eliminate the negative, latch on to the affirmative . . ." or, "Smile though your heart is breaking . . . smile even though it's aching . . ." I once asked Grandma how she managed to get through the death of so many important people in her life, including two husbands. "I don't think, *I lost them*," she replied. "I think, *I had them*."

Every day I remind myself that I don't have to be a cynical bitch, even when the world perplexes me. I admit that I don't always succeed, but the more I allow myself to let go, the more fulfillment I find. And just as with the weight I wore on my stomach, the emotional weight that goes with hanging on to anger doesn't serve me, even though it protects me, or rather, gives the illusion of protecting me.

So if food does not rule my life, what does? I could be

codependent and say that my marriage does, but that wouldn't be entirely accurate. My marriage to Mariann gives me companionship, camaraderie, and a quirky and brilliant compatriot with whom I can explore this world and this life. My marriage does not rule me, though. I would venture to guess that if it did, it would be a pretty lackluster partnership.

And though it's frequently the reason I jump out of bed in the morning, my awareness of animal suffering does not define or rule my life, either. It gives me an important reason to stay focused, to stay passionate, and it allows me the great gift of having a much-bigger-than-me purpose. But it doesn't rule me.

What rules me is possibility. What rules me is the knowledge, firsthand, that people change, that society as a whole shifts, and that empathy is perhaps innate—even though it often becomes misplaced, or snowed under. What rules me is the awareness that even though I feel I have gravitated toward compassion in ways that were once so foreign to me, there are so many other forms of oppression that I don't yet know about, and it humbles me to think that I'm still evolving. I will always be evolving. I wonder what's next. I wonder how my life will change as new truths become clear to me. (And I wonder what my hair will look like then.)

It's easy to get complacent and ignore the issues in this world . . . *or* . . . we can do whatever is in our power to change it. For me, that shift was not fully possible until I first changed myself. I needed to find my truth.

I needed to find my juicer.

Mariann and I are headed out to the theater. Tonight, we are going to see the revival of *Cabaret*, one of Mariann's favorites—she has always had a fondness for theatrical productions with political themes. It's past seven—so we are officially running late.

"Honey, we've gotta go," says Mariann, as she roams throughout the apartment, searching in various corners for her black pleather oxfords. (Between the two of us, we have quite a collection of these, and lucky for us, we wear the same shoe size. #lesbianperks)

I look up at the mirror, adjust my necklace, press my lips together to even out my gloss. And even though we are going to be late and I really don't have time for this, I linger for an extra few moments on my reflection.

"Hello," I say to the woman staring back at me in the mirror. "It's nice to meet you." A moment later I add, "I'm Jazz."

"Did you say something?" asks Mariann from the bedroom.

"Nope," I lie, continuing to look at this veritable stranger in front of me and inside of me.

The woman in the mirror stares back. I question her motives and squint my eyes a little. "What do you want?" I asked quietly, wondering if I have finally fallen off my rocker.

What *do* I want?

The ultimate irony is staring me in the face: When I was fat, in many ways I knew exactly who I was—I was used to the girl, then the woman, in the mirror staring back. While it was true that I wasn't comfortable in my body, it turned out I was very comfortable in my character. I knew my talents and I felt solid in my strengths. When I lost the weight, and my physical appearance became something I was recognized for—and not in a negative way, for the first time in my life—everything became a bit off-kilter, and for a long time I struggled, unable to find inner balance.

Once I started to recognize that I was suddenly reaping the benefits of arbitrary perks—and it concurrently sank in that these perks were the flip side of the bullying and invalidation I had been living with my whole fat life—I began to second-guess everybody's motives. If somebody asked me to tell them about my work, for example, a part of me wondered if they would have bothered inquiring had I been a hundred pounds heavier. I would reply, of course, but there was all too often now a jaded cynicism underlying my perfectly polite response.

The irony that crystalized was startling: Although as a fat person I was oppressed by a society that eagerly cast me aside, as a thin person, I oppressed myself with my doubts and my second thoughts. As a thin person, I could no longer make sense of my life as I knew it. It was like I was coming up in the world again, starting from scratch.

I take a tiny, self-defensive step away from the mirror, but continue to look. I am momentarily startled by how straight I am standing. The lone long piece of my asymmetrical short hair—sprinkled each day with more and more silver—falls in a determined chunk onto my face. I wear bright blue cat-eye glasses—beneath them, my hazel eyes are rimmed with what might very well be a little too much black liner (some habits die hard). A small nose hoop catches the dim light.

I notice that I look more serious than I used to, evident from my hint of a furrowed brow, which suddenly seems to be as permanently a part of me as my tattoos.

But my reflection in the mirror carries an unmistakable hopefulness, too—a determination to continue to seek the truth in the world and in myself, a baseline understanding that change is always possible, even though it might sometimes be seen, at first anyway, as radical. I am no longer full of desperation—four tiny syllables that managed to define my life for so long. Of course, I don't have all the answers yet, but I do have an unrelenting determination to keep trying to figure them out.

When my grandmother was dying, Mariann and I sat at her bedside for eight days, along with our dog, Rose, and my mother and stepfather. Grandma struggled to hang on, a devastating and deeply moving process that will haunt me forever. As Grandma moaned in what was undoubtedly the knowledge that these were her final days—moments she did not want to let go of—Mariann, who was my strength, too, in that dark time, would hold Grandma's hand and gently stroke her cheek, saying repeatedly, "You are doing everything right. You are exactly where you should be."

You are exactly where you should be. It is something Grandma used to say to me, though I never quite believed it. This idea that I'm exactly where I should be—which is something that I regularly try to remind myself, now that Grandma isn't around—helps me face, and even embrace, my powerlessness when confronted with a seemingly untenable situation. If I can get myself to accept that I am indeed precisely where I need to be, it can ground me—and so it has been a mantra sporadically peppered throughout my life. In the depths of any despair, finding—or even just seeking—that kind of validation can be liberating.

I continue to stare at my reflection, no longer worrying about the time. I quietly sing the line, "You're so vain . . ." and I step a little bit farther back from the mirror. If it weren't for my tattoos, I'm not sure I would know this is me. My body is strong—the muscles on my legs defined and ready. I am wearing a simple, form-fitting, sleeveless black dress, dark tights, and gold-toed oxfords (I keep refusing to let Mariann borrow this pair). There is a ring on nearly each of my fingers—but the one that strikes me the most in this moment is my simple wedding band, which I delicately touch with my thumb.

As I look fixatedly at myself, my gaze stops at my stomach. I am reminded that my massive weight loss has left a lumpy and misshapen middle, but nothing that strategically chosen clothes can't hide. Still, it seems an unfair side effect of reclaiming my health and my sense of self. I touch the "problem area," then frown, cock my head, and—surprising myself—simply shrug. "Big deal," I whisper so quietly that the whole world would have to turn down its volume for anyone to hear.

This person in the mirror, this is someone I know, though not entirely. She is someone I am beginning to understand, am just starting to *get*.

And she is indeed exactly as she is supposed to be.

ACKNOWLEDGMENTS

I wish I could publish an entire sequel to this book that is just for acknowledgments. I feel like the luckiest person in the world, to know—and to have known—the people whose names you are about to read. And I'm probably also the shittiest person in the world, because I will undoubtedly forget many, and I will surely kick myself time and time again for those people I foolishly left out of these pages. So let me first thank those very people whom I carelessly left out of this section. If that's you, then please know how much you mean to me, and how vitally important your support has been at one time or another throughout my life, culminating in this book—which simply would not have been possible without you.

Even though I practically ripped apart the bulk of my adolescence in the preceding pages, there were very important forces in my life at that time that encouraged my talents and kept me more or less sane. These include Jodi Antinori ("Ms. McBride"), Jacqueline Geiger, Elaine Koplow, Gil Burgess, Angela DeCandia Ermi, Peter Catenacci, Charlie Gilbert, Leigh Smiley-Grace, Barb Martin, Ruis Woertendyke, and Chris Thomas. I kind of think it's possible I wouldn't be alive without each of you. I am also extremely grateful for the positive impact that Clara Varlese and Emily Calabrese had on my college years, simply by being true to yourselves.

And, Brock Haussamen, thank you for always being so gentle and kind. Maybe you now know how important you were, and how that small chunk of time when we were family forever changed me for the better.

Thanks to James Cunningham for all those Coffee Coolattas, and for all that priceless love, which has very much shaped me (and perhaps continues to).

I owe a gigantic amount of debt to my family—both the one I was born into and the one I married into. Kit Klauss, Gerd Klauss, Patrick Klauss, Anna Dalla Val, Julia Klauss, Sienna Klauss, Christina Spieler, Russ Spieler, Max Sullivan Spieler, Grayson Spieler, and Anne Schneider—I am so happy to know each of you. Thank you for the support you have offered me with the publication of my book.

Thanks to my brilliant and bold niece, Lila Fay Singer, for always reminding me that it's completely appropriate to assert yourself when you want to be heard. And thanks to her parents, Hilary Cohen Singer, whom I would have chosen as my sister if I'd had that option (but I'm so happy that it happened anyway), and Jeremy Singer, my big brother, for always being in my corner, even when neither of us are being overt about that (I'm in your corner, too). Thanks to Jordana Reim, Aviva Reim, Bruce Reim, and Maia Reim, for the silliness, and for the precious familial bond.

I am so totally grateful to Wayne Omohundro, my patient and unwavering stepfather. Your first gift to me was a porcelain clown doll, which still sits in my bedroom. But it's the thousands of gifts you've given me since then that have helped shape the person I am today, and I am certain I would be a shell of myself without your quiet but consistent love. I'm truly sorry that I was such a bitch to you for the entirety of my childhood. You have always been so reliable and generous, and you have never asked for anything in return.

(Mom, please don't panic. I promise I will thank you before the book is done.)

My friends have been my family, too, and my story would be colorless without them. Thank you to my earliest connections: Patricia Craig (you will always be Patty Fonseca to me), Sonia Ahluwalia Khanna, Tamika Langley, Bonnie Smith, Lauren Hasinger, Jessica Sarnicola, and all the other kids who didn't make fun of me. (Actually, thanks to the ones who did make fun of me, too. Though I do really wish you hadn't, I guess I'm more interesting today because of my scars.)

Huge thanks to my darling friends of the present day, including David Williams (I . . . you), Sara Leavitt (I think of you every time I put on purple eye shadow!), Jane Hoffman, Ellen Celnik, Beth Greenfield, Kiki Herold, Angie Lovell, Josh Hanagarne, Donna Dennison, Rachel Duvall, Amy Trakinski, Angie Lovell, Derek Goodwin, Kara Davis, Paula Burke, John Yunker, Lucy Wainwright Roche, Maya Lahr Gottfried, Elisa Camahort Page, Gretchen Primack, Michelle Rubin, Lynn Chen, Sally Tamarkin, Michelle Schwegmann, Josh Hooten, Meena Alagappan, Robert Friedlander, Kerrie Ann Murphy, Debbie Cravey, Beth Lyons, Kerry Lea, Aviv Roth, Patrick Kwan, Jo-Anne McArthur, Liz Marshall, Mia MacDonald, Laura Handzel, Pam Frasch, Debbie Walker, Marisa Miller Wolfson, David Wolfson, Jessica Mahady, Michelle Carrera, Ollie Carrera, and Blythe Ann Boyd. Thanks to my fabulous friends Ethan Ciment and Michael Suchman, who constantly fill my heart and my stomach. Thanks to Jane Velez-Mitchell for making sure I was writing when I was supposed to be, and for always saying it like it is. Thanks to Martin Rowe for giving me stupendous advice on writing and running (and writing about running) for so many years. Thanks to Scott Spitz and the entire Strong Hearts Vegan Power running community (if you're going to be stuck in a van with anyone, it might as well be them).

Thanks to my heroes in the animal rights movement, including many of the people I just mentioned, as well as Gene Baur, Matt Ball, Brad Goldberg, Wayne Pacelle, Kathy Freston, Dr. Neal Barnard, Susie Coston, Steve Wise, Nathan Runkle, Jenny Brown, Doug Abel, Kim Sturla, Ingrid Newkirk, Kathy Stevens, Matt Rice, Paul Shapiro, James McWilliams, Laura George, Ariel Nessel, Alissa Hauser, and Miriam Jones. Thanks, too, to Dr. Robert Ostfeld, Dr. Joel Fuhrman, and Joe Cross, for influencing me in my journey, and for shedding a much-needed light on the awesome health benefits of plants. Thanks to my tap dance community, especially Tony Waag and the American Tap Dance Foundation, Laura Pearson, whose advice and friendship are as nourishing as her homemade vegan cheese, and Barbara Duffy, whom I look up to so much, and whose talent and insight are equally unsurpassed. And a shout-out to the rest of the Thursday Girls—Crystal Love Tiffany, Deb Pelton Hall, and Tina Micic, for tapping it out with me.

My dear soul-friends, Alexander Gray and David Cabrera, are true heroes and besties. Thank you for letting me use your house to write, your ears to vent, your shoulders to cry on, and your wisdom to guide me. I feel lucky every single day to have you in my life. (Even though you somehow make me buy knives and houses that were never in the budget.) I completely love you both.

My heart is full when I think of the many healers I've had throughout my life, and those include Brett Kennedy, Guy Winch, Susan M. MacKinnon, and Jane E. Gartner. Special thanks to J. D. Davids for the gentle guidance, and for being a role model.

Gena Hamshaw and Victoria Moran were like little guideposts during the early days of writing this book, and I am so very appreciative. You are both mentors of mine, and I'm so grateful that you so generously shared your resources and your experiences while I was first putting pen to paper. Nell Alk, I'm pretty sure that this book would not exist if you didn't strongly encourage me to publish my article about my shifting perceptions of the world from losing weight, and if you didn't proactively introduce me to *MindBodyGreen*. I owe you so much. And thank you to *MindBodyGreen*, too, for finding a home for my article "What Losing 100 Pounds Taught Me about How We Treat Overweight People." Special thanks to those who provided feedback on early drafts of my manuscript, including bob McNeil (my sandbox buddy for life), and Rhona Melsky.

Thanks to my amazingly talented editor, Allison Janice, for believing in me from the get-go, and for discovering and then pursuing this project. I felt safe with you and trusted your judgment with my manuscript, even when the track changes made me want to kill myself. I am so grateful. And thanks to everyone at Berkley for working with me on this—I couldn't have asked for a better team. I'm very thankful, too, to my incredible agent, Steve Troha, from Folio Literary Management, and to Dado

Derviskadic, for holding my hand when I needed it, and for showing me how to find my wings. You're the best on earth. Steve, your advice to get off my soapbox whenever I felt I was beginning to proselytize was, even in its simplicity, groundbreaking for me (even though I didn't always succeed). Thanks, too, to my publicity team at The Tasc Group.

The Our Hen House community is what keeps me going, day in and day out, and so thank you from the bottom of my heart to my podcast listeners, TV show viewers, flock members, and many amazing supporters for all the love you have given to me and Mariann since day one, and for being so passionate about changing the world for animals. A huge gigantic thanks to Anne Green for reading the first incarnation of my manuscript and providing me with such valuable feedback, and for always e-mailing to me "Never fear!" at exactly the right moment. Thanks to Alessandra Seiter for constantly impressing me with your incredible skills, and for always making me think longer and harder. Thanks to Ben Braman, Eric Milano, Danielle Legg, and Laurie Johnston. And thanks to my amazing board of directors and their partners: Liz Dee and Nick Garin, J. L. Fields and Dave Burgess, Alison Mercer and Kevin Mercer, and, of course, the aforementioned Michael and Ethan, and Alex and David. Thanks to our wonderful writers, reviewers, and volunteers, including Ari Solomon, Robin Lamont, Ken Swensen, Piper Hoffman, Cassandra Greenwald, Bonnie Goodman, Michael Harren, and Keri Cronin. A very special thank you to Kathy Head, and additional thanks to the awesome team over at Brooklyn Independent Media.

(Don't worry, Mom. I promise I haven't forgotten about you.)

Thanks to my childhood (and, ahem, adulthood) idols, Patti LuPone and Bette Midler, who have been turning me into a puddle for twenty-five years. When I was a kid, you showed me that it was okay to be an oddball, as long as you were a driven one.

There are those who are no longer with us to whom I'm eternally grateful. My sweet grandpa, Murray Glickman, who constantly thought my jokes were hilarious (even when they weren't); Muriel Alpern, for the cat tchotchkes, and for always reading (and liking) my poetry; George Reim, for being such a legendary guy—I wish I had known you; and my childhood cat, Rocky, for proving that there's always a way out when you want there to be, as long as you're determined. (Thanks, too, for always coming back home to me.)

An enormous thank-you to Rose Singer-Sullivan, my precious, beautiful, sweet, cozy, silly, sensitive dog. Rose is a gentle and loving pit bull who was found tied to a pole, where she had been left for several days. At just one year old, she had just weaned puppies, and most likely was being used as a breeding dog for an illegal operation. She was taken to a "shelter," where at the time they killed all pit bulls, but an "underground railroad" of sorts, created by loving employees, snuck Rose out and into a loving home. Rose has taught me that it is possible to trust again, and to love wholly and unconditionally. She kept me company for many hours, days, weeks, and months while this book was being written, and I'm sure it wouldn't have been if she wasn't right beside me throughout.

Okay, Mom, here comes your part: I know you have not always had it easy, having me as your daughter, and I know that there were many other aspects of your own life that were challenging, too. But we've worked it out somehow, and I am so beholden to you for all you have given to me, but mostly, for always believing in me. Thank you for attending each one of my shows, reading my many hundreds of stories and poems, and always sharing my Facebook statuses on your page with a cute little doting comment. I look up to you for always being so strong, loyal, and creative, and I'm proud to be your daughter. Roni Omohundro, I promise my next book will only say wonderful things about you.

This book was dedicated to my grandmother, Sherrey Reim Glickman, and I just want to reiterate my extreme gratitude to her. Grandma was, in so many ways, my heartbeat, and now the echo of her heartbeat courses through me. She always told me I'd be a writer, even when that annoyed me and I insisted that, no, I'd be an actress. She was exceptional, and I hope that in my life I can be half as poised as she was.

Finally, I want to thank my wife, Mariann Sullivan. For nearly a decade, you have been by my side for better or for worse, and you have stuck with me even when I was absolutely impossible to deal with. You woke up at six A.M. to edit my book, you dragged your ass to Red Hook, Brooklyn, to watch me workshop an undeveloped scene from these pages (even though you were forced to do a weird theater exercise), you gently corrected me when I was using adjectives incorrectly, and you consistently praised me when I doubted myself—but never so much that it went to my head. You have been my rock and my guide, my partner in life and my very best friend. This book is, in so very many ways, because of you, and my love for you is all encompassing. I will work until the end of my days to do my best to deserve you, and to make you feel as safe as you make me feel.